Sudden Vision

The "RK" Procedure for Nearsightedness
and Other Wonders of
Modern Ophthalmology

by John Crater
Cartoons by Bud Root and John Crater
Illustrations by Herb King

Consultants:
Marvin J. Grendahl, M.D.
James J. Salz, M.D.
Leo D. Bores, M.D.

SLACK Inc. 6900 Grove Road Thorofare NJ 08086

Please read this first!

This book contains no instructions for any kind of operation or treatment. All medical decisions must be based on your doctor's advice and your own desires. The author is not an authority, does not have any professional expertise or financial interest in these procedures, and wishes merely to throw some light to help you find the safest path to your goal.

"RK", the operation for nearsightedness (poor distance vision) that is the main subject of this book, has been a fantastic opportunity for some patients. But is RK a good idea for you?

Sudden Vision will not answer that question. It will help you to answer it yourself, by helping you to understand this extraordinary subject so that you can discuss it with your doctor as one informed person talking to another.

To Mom and Dad

Copyright © 1990 by John Crater

All rights reserved. No part of this book may be reproduced, stored in a retrieval system or transmitted in any form or by any means, electronic, mechanical, photocopying, recording or otherwise, without written permission from the copyright holder, except for brief quotations embodied in critical articles or reviews.

Printed in the United States of America

Library of Congress Catalog Card Number: 89-042918

ISBN: 1-55642-123-0

Published by: SLACK Incorporated
6900 Grove Road
Thorofare, NJ 08086

Copies of this book are available to ophthalmologists and optometrists from SLACK Inc.

This book is also distributed (to all others) by
Useful Publishing
P.O. Box 242244
Anchorage AK 99524-2244

A Sudden Change in Your Vision?

If you wear glasses or contacts and would rather not, today's ophthalmology may offer you a way to get rid of them. You have probably heard of the "RK" operation, which consists of shallow incisions in the outer part of the cornea, the front window of the eye. This operation, which has already helped about 250,000 nearsighted Americans (including the author), has excellent odds of success for ordinary nearsightedness.

People with severe myopia, astigmatism and even farsightedness can also benefit from new techniques in the amazing field of "refractive surgery". All eyewear-dependent Americans should be aware of the revolution in vision care that is taking place in this country.

Sudden Vision tackles such questions as:
What are my chances of coming away with 20/20?
How can I maximize my chances of success?
Does the operation hurt? How many days of work would I miss?
Does it take effect immediately?
How do I find the best surgeon to perform my operation?
Will my insurance pay for it?
What are the risks and drawbacks? How can I minimize them?
What about the mid-life vision change, when people usually start wearing reading glasses or bifocals—does this affect my RK planning?
Will RK help me join the police/ fire department/ armed forces?
Can my children avoid nearsightedness?

Your eyes have read a thousand books for you—read one book for them!

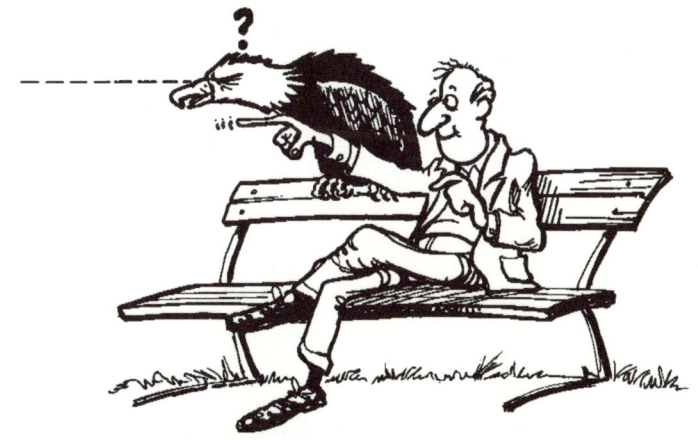

Contents

Foreword by Dr. Leo D. Bores
1. Suddenly, an Alternative 1
2. The Infinite Inch 11
3. Optalk: Measuring Refraction 23
4. Hey Strong-Eyes! 29
5. How RK Does It 41
6. You Can't Cram for a Pre-RK Exam 49
7. Two Eyes, Two Visions 59
8. The RK Candidate Plans the Campaign 69
9. The RK Operation 79
10. Sight for Sore Eye: the RK Recovery 87
11. But Does It Work? Results of RK 95
12. Potential Problems with RK 105
13. The RK Decision:
    It's Great to Have a Choice 117
14. "Blind Without Glasses"? Not Forever! 129
15. Another Ism We Could Do Without 139
16. Finding the Doc and the Dollars 147
17. We'll All Have 20/20 by 2020 159

Appendices:
   A. This Has Gone Farsighted Enough 171
   B. Two Cheers for Glasses & Contact Lenses ... 179
   C. Eyemergencies 189
   D. RK Checklist 199

Glossary 201
Index 209
Acknowledgements 214
About this Edition 215

Foreword

Here at last is a guide to "RK" and the other new vision alternatives that's genuinely fun to read, with hundreds of illustrations and cartoons. The author's explanations of complicated subjects are such a pleasure that I intend to steal—ah, borrow—some of them in my talks with my own patients. In fact, anyone who is considering refractive surgery should read *Sudden Vision*. The reader will come away with an understanding of this fascinating matter, and with confidence, enthusiasm, and the ability to participate fully in the process.

The field of refractive surgery is growing rapidly. It now has much to offer those who long for improved vision, and it will continue to offer more with each passing year. The prospects for astigmatic and farsighted people are very exciting, and Mr. Crater has taken the trouble to include these developments and a great deal of other information never brought under one roof before. And there are chapters on contact lenses and eye emergencies that everybody should read.

Electing to have one of these small but powerful operations is a serious personal decision and not well illuminated by media hype or advertising, yet in the past that's about all there was to introduce the average person to our field of ophthalmology. This book changes that: a realistic understanding of these new alternatives is now available to anyone.

Sudden Vision is also recommended reading for the ophthalmologist, providing insights not otherwise obtainable—and from someone who has "been there".

                              Leo D. Bores, M.D.
                              Scottsdale, Arizona April 14, 1988

Suddenly, an Alternative

The change was sudden and startling. The doctor untaped the patch that I had worn over my right eye since the operation the day before, and slowly I opened the eye and gazed at the world with 20/20 vision. I knew that it would be several days at least before the final result would be known, but it was looking good.

Like hundreds of thousands of other Americans I had undergone refractive surgery, a subspecialty of ophthalmology (eye surgery) that improves the focusing, or refraction, of the patient's eyes. My operation, "RK" for nearsightedness and mild astigmatism, is the most widely available of the new procedures. Others are being developed to help people with farsightedness and even presbyopia, the loss of near vision in middle age.

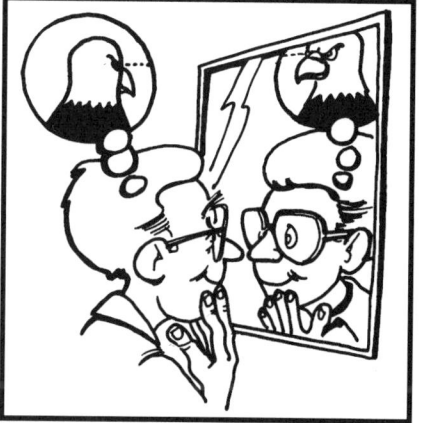

If you are nearsighted you're one of at least eighty million such Americans; without us they couldn't run this country for a week. We are strong citizens and in fact that's the nature of our visual problem: our eyes have too much focusing power. We're strong-eyed.

Nearsightedness, or myopia, does have its bright side. We tend to be well-educated, successful people. We're great at tying fishooks. And we get a consolation prize: the same surplus eyepower that blurs our distance vision also provides close-up vision in the post-40 half of life, when our 20/20 friends all need reading glasses.

In every other respect nearsightedness is an unmitigated nuisance. To see clearly we have to wear lenses, either saddled across the nose or afloat in the tear film. We're stereotyped by fools and discriminated against by bureaucracies.

A Major Minority

Has the time come for Nearsighted Liberation? "All Power to the Strong-Eyes!" we could cry from the barricades. "Up against the wall, bare-eyes!" Considering the discrimination we endure, it's a pity we're too diverse and individualistic to start a Front. We're a polyglot crew, millions of one-of-a-kind people with all degrees of myopia (nearsightedness). Many also have astigmatism to complicate things. We live in every country and belong to both sexes and all races. We deal with the problem in many different ways and wear all kinds of glasses and contact lenses.

Most of us do have one thing in common: a misunderstanding of what's really going on with our eyes. We don't understand why we're nearsighted, why our children become nearsighted, or what the consequences of nearsightedness are as the midlife vision change begins to unfold. We don't know that we're at higher risk of detached retinas. We may know how powerful the lenses are in our field glasses and cameras, but we often don't know the same detail about our own eyes, and can't read our own eyeglass prescriptions. And most nearsighted people don't know about the new way of relieving nearsightedness, the new micro-operation called Radial Keratotomy (or RK).

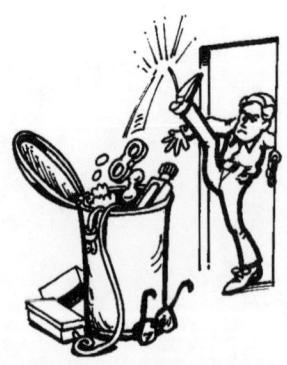

Seeing is Believing

I had RK in 1985, and it was one of the most amazing experiences of my life. A quarter century of being nearsighted (and hating it) was suddenly over. If done in the right way by the right doctor on the right person, RK can be sensational.

After the operation, my friends would ask why I wasn't wearing glasses. I would explain how my glasses had been surgically removed. That raised some eyebrows! Some of them had terrible misconceptions about RK—that it was desperately risky, or only done in Europe—but most had never even heard of it.

The Third Alternative

Until recently, progress in treating nearsightedness was glacially slow. For thousands of years, nearsighted people just squinted and made fist-pinholes and tried to get by. Only in this millenium did glasses become available—although for a long time they were believed to cause blindness! In the last half-century, a second alternative appeared: the contact lens. Most eye professionals were shocked at first by the idea of a foreign object deliberately left in the eye—unlike glasses, this really could cause blindness. But eventually it became clear that the risks were acceptable to many people who were unhappy with glasses.

And for the past ten years, RK has presented a third, very different and exciting approach: built-in, non-prosthetic, a permanent improvement in the shape of the eye. An actual cure, instead of a device. It began in Japan, was resurrected in Moscow, but has now become predominantly an American operation. American ophthalmologists—eye-specializing MD's—have developed the specialized instruments, improved the techniques, published scores of papers and articles, and otherwise completely taken the lead in this new field. Over a quarter of a million RK procedures have been done in the U.S.A.

RK is not a sure thing. About 90% of the people who try it are able to stop wearing glasses or at least have their nearsightedness so greatly decreased that they're happy. There's no way to be sure you'll emerge a perfect 20/20, but this book will show you the steps you can take to improve the odds of success.

Glasses-Wearers of the World, Rejoice

People with farsightedness and astigmatism should also learn about the new alternatives now becoming available. Ophthalmologists are developing methods of permanently correcting all of the common focusing errors. Even "presbyopia", the loss of close-up focusing that occurs after age 40, may soon be helped by refractive surgery.

These errors in focusing, called "refractive errors", are not complex or mysterious. They're as simple as a home-movie screen set too far back from the projector, so that the picture is out of focus. Mother Nature runs the show, with an iron hand—you're not allowed to move the screen up closer, and you're not allowed to focus the projector! With RK and the other procedures that are called refractive surgery, the surgeon *does* focus the projector, by adjusting the focal power of the round, clear front window of the eye—that bit of human optics called the cornea.

What You *Do* Know can Help You Plenty

Most of this book is useful to anyone who values their eyes, but it was written especially for nearsighted people who want to learn about RK. It's fortunate that nearsightedness has always been associated with a love of learning and self-improvement, because no other operation depends so much on the patient's self-education and participation.

This book will tell you RK's potential for a person with eyes like yours. You'll learn how to determine whether you can get good vision by having only one eye corrected, as the author did, or whether you'll need to have them both done. You'll understand the surprising drawback to having 20/20 vision in both eyes, the phenomenon that could be called the "revenge of the nearsighted".

If you are younger than 40 or 45, you probably wonder what reading glasses are all about and whether you'll need them. All you have to know is your eyeglasses prescription to know what the midlife vision change will mean to you, and how the way your RK is planned affects your vision later in life.

If you are considering RK, this book will give you the total understanding you need to make the right decisions, and get the most out of this amazing new opportunity.

Let the Children Know!

The widespread ignorance of RK's potential is especially unfair to nearsighted children. We forget how tough being a "four-eyes" can be for kids: the old "I'm-gonna-be-an-astronaut-but-you-can't" taunt, the fact that nearsightedness is a permanent defect, not something temporary like acne or braces. It's even worse now than when we baby-boomers were kids—at least we didn't have to deal with this national obsession with the "nerd", the pitiful, ugly, out-of-it kid who always wears glasses. Since nearsighted kids are probably smarter and more determined than others, this must be the stupidest as well as the cruellest stereotype of them all. Let's get the word to the kids that nearsightedness no longer has to be a permanent condition. Although kids can't have RK, they enjoy knowing they may have a 20/20 future—and that by the time they're our age glasses will probably be considered a temporary nuisance.

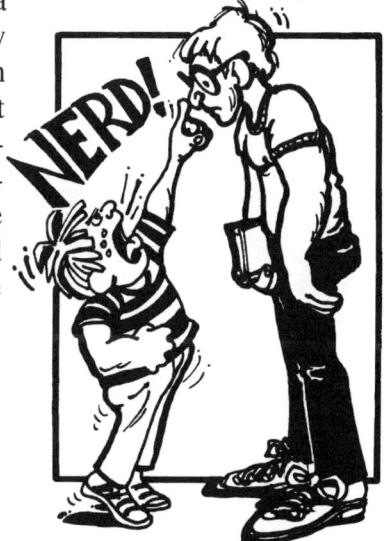

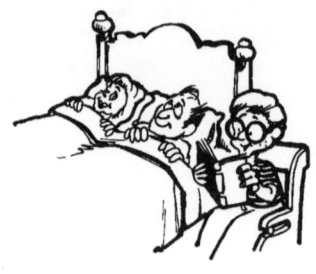

In fact, as we'll see, many nearsighted people can use RK to become better off than if they had 20/20 vision to begin with—they can avoid needing reading glasses in their senior years.

We'll also be examining the possibility that nearsightedness can be prevented, a development every parent should be aware of. And anyone involved with children should read the Appendix on eye emergencies.

Bonus: Be Well Eyeducated

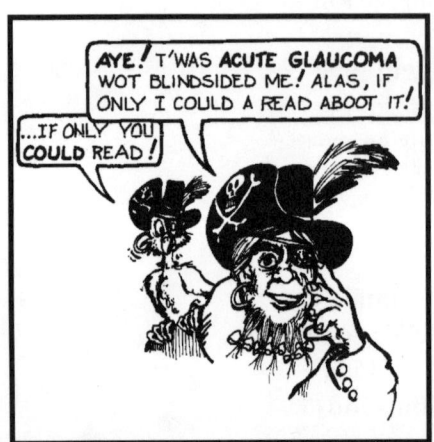

Besides giving you the whole story on permanent focus correction, this book is an owner's manual to your eyes. It doesn't just fill you in on modifications you can make, it also tells you what the heck you already have. The First Aid pages in the back are must-read material for everybody. Having read this book, you'll never again be ignorant and apprehensive about your eyes—you'll be confident and knowledgeable about these tools that you use 18 hours a day.

RK Preview

We are going to examine Radial Keratotomy in complete detail, concentrating on the areas where knowledge can enable you to make a real difference in your chances of success. But right now let's run through the RK process briefly just to get an overview of the subject.

With nearsightedness (also called myopia) the eye has too much focusing power, so the image is focused before it reaches the back of the eye—which means that the image is out of focus again when it strikes the retina, the layer of light-receptor cells that coats the inside of the whole back of the eye.

RK works by making the cornea—the clear, round, curved front window of the eye—a little less strongly curved, thereby allowing the eye to focus more perfectly. Since the cornea is in the very front of the eye and the cuts go only partway through it, the surgery is very fast and superficial. Don't let that fool you, though—a lot is happening in those few minutes. The result will be striking, and usually permanent, and how happy you are about it depends partly on how well you and your doctor make a number of large and small decisions, and how well you do your part as a patient.

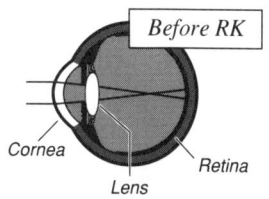

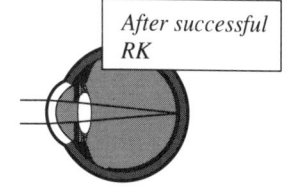

The first thing the prospective patient should do is learn about his or her vision, and RK. You're already off to a strong start on that!

The next step is to choose a qualified ophthalmologist—there's an upcoming chapter to help with that one. Next comes a little thing that is always worth doing, whether you go any further or not: visiting your chosen doctor for a complete eye exam.

About a tenth of nearsighted people will not "pass" this exam, and will either have to wait awhile before going ahead, or be told they're just not a good candidate for some reason. The other 90% will be able to have RK if they desire it, but the prospects for complete success will be brighter for some than for others, depending on such factors as degree of nearsightedness, astigmatism, and age. (Surprisingly, older can be better.)

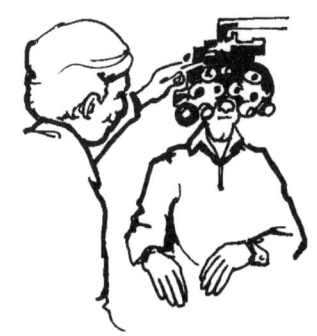

Next Step: the Decision

The great thing about the RK decision is that it is such a leisurely choice—there's no need to hurry, nothing to be lost by waiting or gained by rushing. Take your time. No one has a stake in it but you.

If your decision is a "go", there is some planning to be done by both the patient and the doctor, working together. RK is a matter of degrees, not an

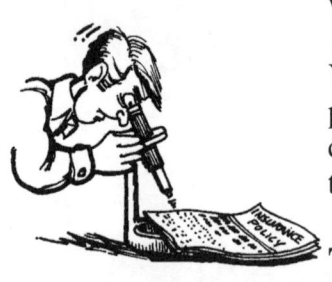

all-or-nothing deal like having your tonsils taken out. If you know just what you want, the doctor will be in a much better position to satisfy you.

There is also the little matter of paying for it. You'll need to check with your insurance company, or make other arrangements. We've included a chapter to help the RK consumer over that hurdle.

The Big Day

Next thing you know, the appointment for the actual operation has arrived. A friend or taxi delivers you to the doctor's surgicenter or office, you take a tranquilizer and relax. The surgery is remarkably painless and untraumatic, with no shots, no blood, no stitches. (And no laser. Sorry.) It takes anywhere from ten minutes to half an hour.

Generally, the eye is very sore for a day, and light-sensitive for a month, and then it's back to normal except for the improvement in vision. But the eye should be protected from unnecessary contamination (or impact) for several weeks, at least. If both eyes are to be done, wait a couple of months before going ahead with the second eye.

Is It Really as Easy as That? No

That sounds simple enough. In fact, however, there are many crucial details which must be understood by the patient who wants to get the greatest benefit from this amazing procedure. Lack of understanding leads patients to make mistakes in choosing whether the surgery is right for them, whether to get both eyes operated on or just one, exactly how much correction the doctor should be trying for in each eye, how to prepare themselves for the surgery, how to get it paid for, and how it should be scheduled. These mistakes cause patients to end up much less satisfied than they could have been, or to miss out on a great opportunity.

RK is very different from other common operations. It isn't intended to stave off some disease or repair some injury, but to produce an astonishing improvement. It can fix something you never thought was fixable. Where other operations are necessary evils, this one is optional, "elective", an unexpected delight. The important thing is to understand it completely, especially the potential problems and shortcomings, and be aware of the steps you will want to take to optimize the results, before you go ahead. There's no excuse for ignorance or misunderstanding when there's no hurry or pressure.

Once in a Lifetime

There are a lot of important and interesting details. Adjusting the focus of one's personal optics is a very unique thing to be doing! Curiously, few of us understand the way our eyes really work, or the change that the eye undergoes as it ages and loses the ability to increase its focusing power for near vision.

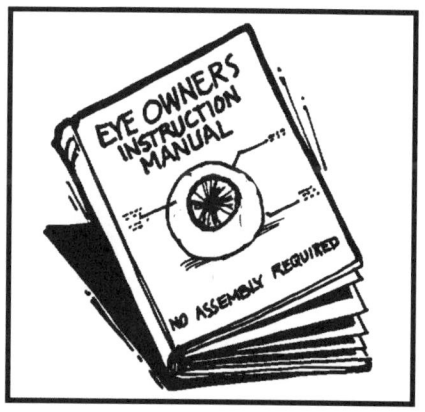

This loss, which the eye doctors call presbyopia but the rest of us call "I need some !*&#!@ reading glasses", is universal. But it means something very different to nearsighted people than it does to the 20/20 folks—because most nearsighted people can still read easily just by taking off their glasses, while the 20/20 types must now wear glasses to read.

This has major implications if you are thinking about becoming a 20/20 type by undergoing RK. There is a way to get the best of both worlds, and need no glasses for distance or for reading, in youth or in old age. It involves having only one eye corrected, with the other eye left alone or only partially corrected. Amazingly, this can often work beautifully if you understand it.

The Jury is In and They're Smiling

RK is still controversal. Some ophthalmologists (including several who've written books) think it's wonderful for nearly all nearsighted folks, and others are flatly against it. But most surgeons who understand RK take a middle view: that it's a very good choice for some people, if both patient and doctor are honest with each other, totally informed, and prepared to do their best to make it a success, even if it means a little more trouble and expense.

After ten years and over 250,000 patients, RK for nearsightedness is a known entity. The advantages and drawbacks of the operation can be spelled out so that each person can make a sound decision, and that is the purpose of this book. I do not perform RK or stand to benefit in any way from promotion of it. I do not care whether you choose RK or not; if you're undecided I'd suggest you hold off. Although RK is great for some people, it's not the right choice for everybody, and only you can decide if it's right for you. I only promise to leave you with a better understanding of your eyes and a better chance of keeping them healthy. And I promise we'll have fun.

Next to see how the little jaspers really work. We're off and running!

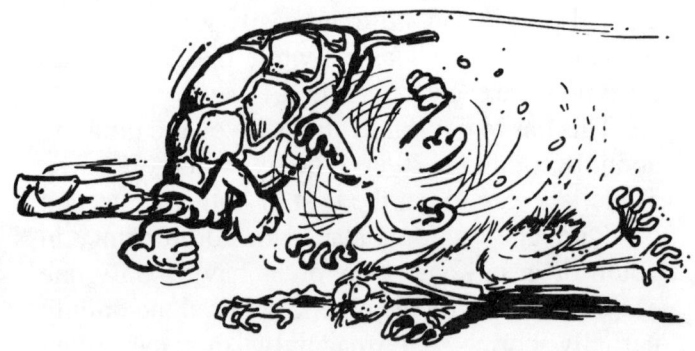

The Infinite Inch 2

The human eye is about one inch in diameter, and must be the most wonderful inch of matter in the known universe. But it's not *quite* perfect.

The eye goes through an unwelcome change beginning around age 40, and failing to understand it can cause serious mistakes in your RK planning. Even if you're just hoping to make the best use of your eyes, let alone trying to improve them through RK, you should understand them as well as a photographer understands his camera.

In fact, the eye is a lot like a camera.

In the front are two transparent bodies that focus light, like a camera's lens. And the whole back half of the eye is covered by the retina, which is light-sensitive like the film in a camera.

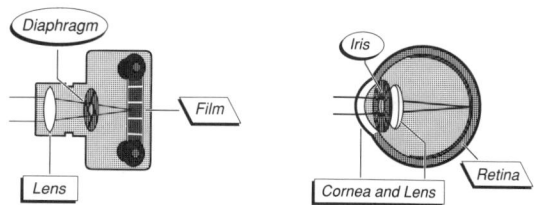

Lens Number One: the Cornea

The front of the eye actually has two lenses to focus light. The first one is the *cornea*, the glassy, curved front window of the eye. The cornea is actually the main lens of the eye, and does about 80% of the focusing.

Behind the cornea is the *iris*, which functions like the diaphragm in a camera. It's actually a little sphincter-type muscle, with some color in it to pretty it up a bit. When it contracts, it shrinks the little hole in the middle called the *pupil*.

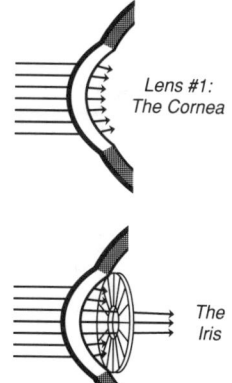

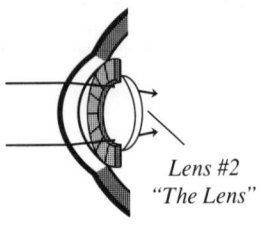
Lens #2 "The Lens"

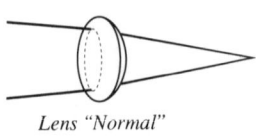
Lens "Normal"

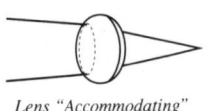
Lens "Accommodating"

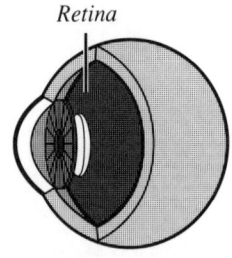
Retina

Lens Number Two: the "Lens"

Just inside the iris is another lens. This one really looks like a lens, and is officially called *the lens*. It's not nearly as strong as the cornea, but it can do something the cornea can't: it can change shape, and *accommodate* for near-point focusing. Until middle age, that is, as we'll discover.

These three components—the cornea, the iris and the lens—are the optical end of the eye, similar to the lens and diaphragm in a camera. They see to it that all light rays from any given point in the field of view get focused upon one corresponding point on the retina.

Brainfilm

The *retina* is a bunch of brain cells in theater seats. They may be like film in a camera, but they're also a kind of audience—about a hundred and forty million silent spectators, munching popcorn and watching whatever visuals you provide. Of course, they only sense light and transmit impulses to the real film buff upstairs, the brain. But in a way they seem to be little brains of their own.

Although the pupil appears dark, actually the inside of your eye is full of light—the whole field of view is being projected on the retina, like a movie on a huge, curving screen. It all gets projected upside down and backwards, but your brain flips it back over for you. If you wear special glasses that turn the view upside down, the brain will re-flip it within a few days.

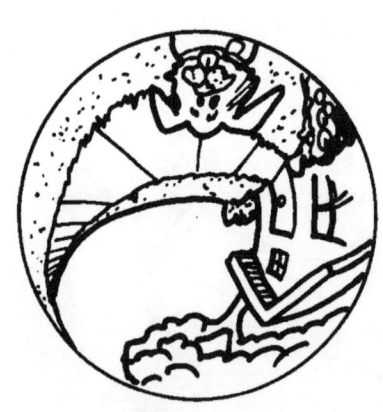

Every point on the retina is being struck by light from one single corresponding point in your field of vision. The lower retina gets the sky, the upper retina gets the ground, the left side sees the view off to the right, and so on.

Here's an everyday scene as it would appear projected on the inside of your eye.

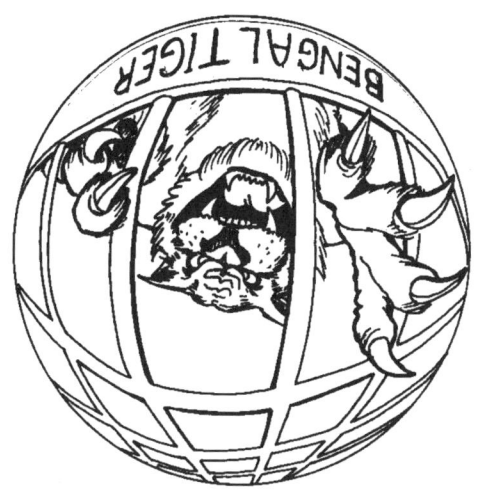

Seeing What You're Looking At

Why is it that only the central part of the field of view is seen distinctly? Because whatever is straight in front of the eye, whatever you are looking directly at, gets projected onto a very special part of the retina. This part of the retina always gets the brain's attention, because there are millions of cells jammed together in a little round patch called the *macula*, and an even more concentrated spot in the center of it called the *fovea*. The light-sensitive retina cells are so packed into this area, and wired so directly to the brain, that they get more attention than all the rest of the retina combined.

The "visual axis" is an imaginary line between whatever you are looking at and the macula/fovea area of your retina. These letters are being projected on that little spot right now!

All the retina cells send messages to the brain through nerve fibers, which join together to form the optic nerve.

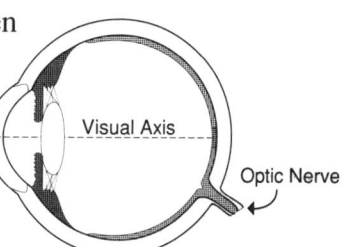

Here's a close-up view of the eye.

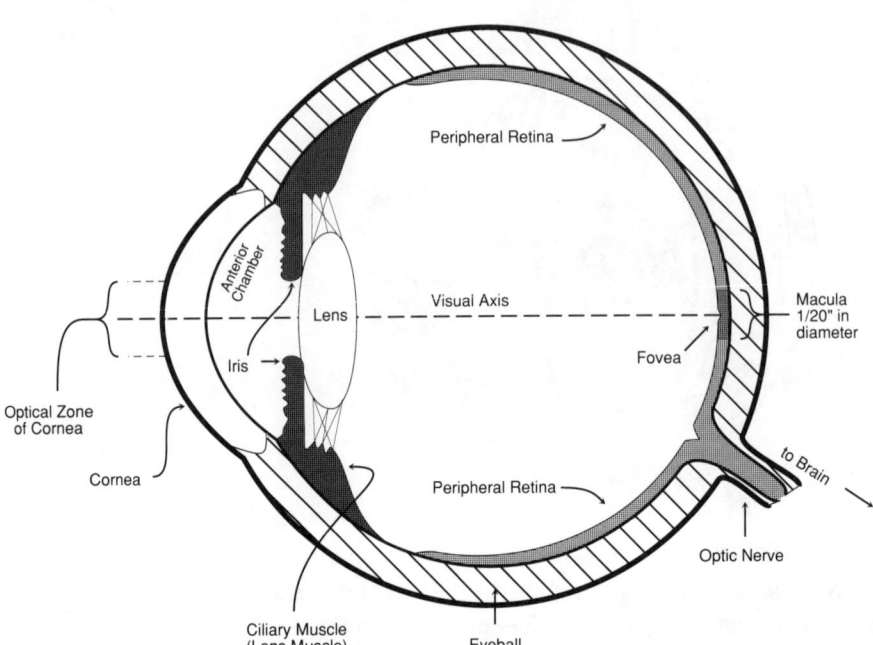

So How Does It Really Work?

How does the light from the world outside the eye, which hits the cornea every which way from all directions, get focused so neatly on the retina? It's only possible because of the law of *refraction*.

Refraction is a word that we'll be using a lot. When an eye doc tests your vision, it's called "taking your refraction". RK is an example of "refractive surgery". Basically, refraction means the bending of light rays as they pass from one clear substance into another. Refraction makes focusing possible, focusing makes vision possible, and vision makes higher life forms possible, so three cheers for refraction!

The Infinite Inch

Physicists call it Snell's Law. For our purposes, this says that the sharper the angle at which light shines into water or glass or the cornea, the more it bends. So if parallel rays of light shine into a convex spherical surface, they get "refracted" together—in other words, focused.

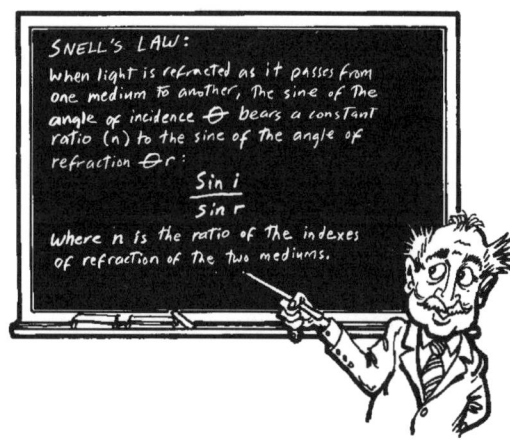

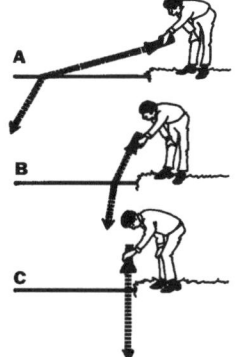

The same principle that makes light bend more as you shine it through water at a sharper angle...

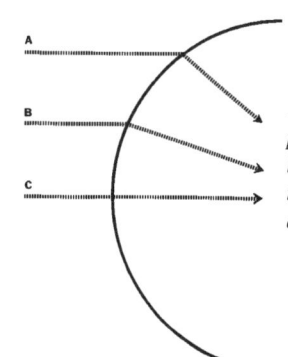

...also makes parallel rays of light focus when they shine through a lens!

Those incoming rays are parallel to each other because they come from the same distant point. This is important: from any point farther than twenty feet away, rays of light strike the eye *virtually parallel* to each other. Imagine how nearly parallel these lines would be if we could move this eye nineteen and a half feet to the right!

So refraction makes parallel light rays bend inward and come to a focus when they enter a spherical surface, like those of your cornea and lens. This is one of physics' niftiest features.

Peripheral vision areas of retina

Macula/Fovea

All the rays from the point you are looking at get focused on the central macula/fovea part of your retina.

Peripheral vision areas of retina

Sudden Vision

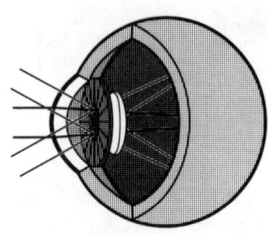

Every point in your view is sending you a set of parallel rays, which get focused on a corresponding point on your retina!

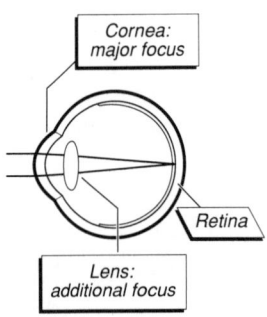

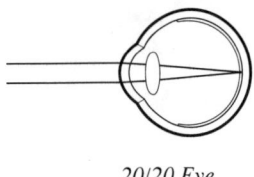

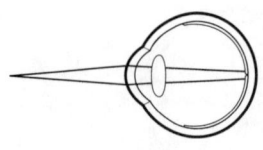

20/20 Eye

Of course, the parallel rays coming in from every other point also get focused—but maybe not quite as well as the rays from straight in front. It's okay if peripheral vision is a little blurry; the brain is mainly concerned with what the macula/fovea area is seeing with its jam-packed millions of receptor cells. Visual-axis vision is what counts.

Refraction in Action

Let's take a closer look at the refraction, or focusing, going on in your eye. The light rays are focused inward by the cornea, and then they are focused even more by the lens.

So the cornea is really a stronger lens than the lens is. But the cornea is rigid and fixed, and can't increase its focusing power: it's not adjustable.

The lens, on the other hand, can be scrunched up into a thicker, rounder shape, thereby increasing its focal power. This is called *accommodation*.

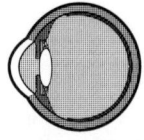 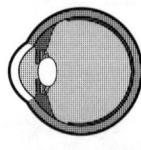

Also, during accommodation, the pupil constricts and the eyes turn inward

Normal   *Accommodated*

Why do you need accommodation? Well, let's assume this eye is perfect—20/20 vision, not nearsighted or farsighted. So all parallel rays striking the cornea from one point in the distance get bent inward and focused exactly on the retina.

But rays from a *near* point are *not* parallel. They diverge as they fan out to all parts of your cornea, or even to all parts of the optical zone over your pupil. This presents a problem.

Because, of course, the same amount of optical power that is just right for focusing parallel rays is not enough to focus these diverging near-point rays. More "bending power" is needed to herd these fanning-out rays in to a single spot on the retina.

The Infinite Inch

Watch the lens do its accommodation routine! Here's distance vision—no problem.

Now you need to see something close. But the near-point rays aren't coming to a focus on your retina.

Your brain tells the eye to make the lens bulge more, which increases its power and bends those rays in a little farther, focusing them nicely. How very accommodating!

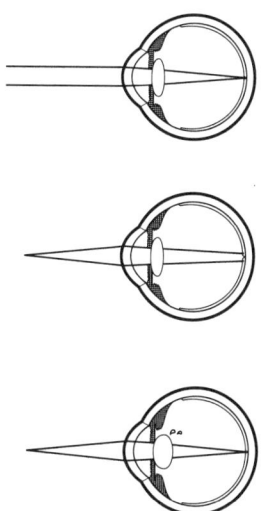

Here's How I Know My Youth is All Spent: My Get-up & Go has Got-up & Went. And so has my Accommodation!

Accommodation is a pretty good trick, but unfortunately it gets lost—the lens stiffens as you get older, until by age 65 you can't accommodate at all.

Children have tremendous accommodation—they can focus on a point just a few inches away. By age 30, you can focus on a point about a foot away. By 40, maybe two feet. By the time you are 45 or fifty, your arms are too short to hold a book far enough away to focus on it!

This loss of near vision is called "presbyopia" (Latin for "old sight") and it happens to everyone—it's so universal that when it doesn't happen, the doc suspects trouble, namely incipient cataracts.

Convex "reading glasses" add positive focusing power—they bend the diverging rays inward, and turn them into parallel distance-type rays.

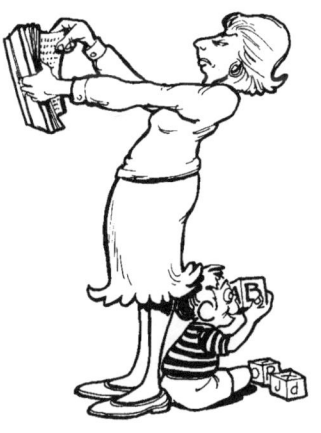

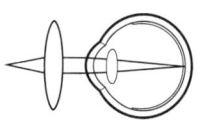

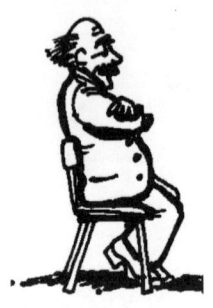

Most people get their first pair of reading glasses or bifocals when they're 40 or 45. They get a new pair with stronger lenses every couple of years until they're about 65. By that age, no accommodation ability remains, and they have full-powered reading glasses. That's complete presbyopia: the lens cannot add any extra power for near-point focusing.

Check Yours

Test your own accommodation ability. Close one eye and hold your thumb about a foot away. Look past it at the background. Your thumb looks blurry, because diverging rays from it are not getting focused enough to meet on your retina.

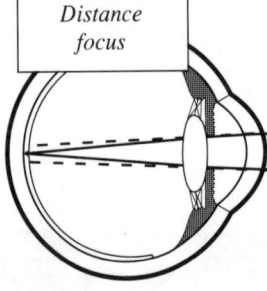

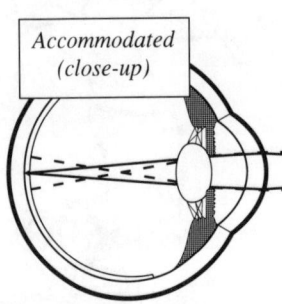

Now focus on your thumb. You can feel your lens' little muscle working! Of course, now the background is blurry, because the parallel distance rays are being focused before they reach the retina.

Accommodation makes it possible to see both near and far out of the same eyes without glasses. Once you lose accommodation, you won't be able to, without reading glasses or bifocals. This is one of the striking design flaws of the human body—cameras handle this better than our eyes do.

With a camera, the lens slides forward, providing more room for the rays to focus for near vision.

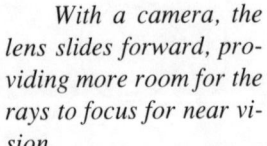
Distance focus

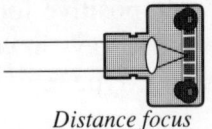

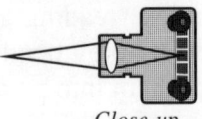
Close-up

Now Let's Get Real

We've been looking at a perfect, "emmetropic" eye that's not farsighted or nearsighted, and we've seen how it changes as it gets older and loses the ability to accommodate. We'll study farsightedness in Appendix A. But most readers are nearsighted folks, who make about a third of the population. (The best third, right?)

Too Strong for Your Own Good: The Nearsighted Eye

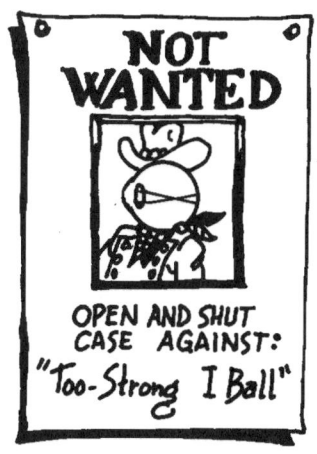

The nearsighted (myopic) eye is too strong—it focuses too much. The image is in focus before it hits the retina; by the time the rays reach the retina they're back out of focus again. Sometimes the cornea is too curved; more often the eyeball is too long. Either way, the result is the same. The cornea won't flatten out...

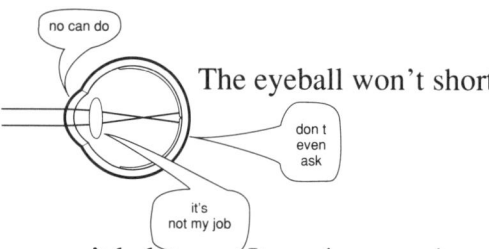

The eyeball won't shorten ...

The lens can't help. It can increase its power, but can't decrease it—can't "anti-accommodate".

What a useless bunch of losers!

So the nearsighted person is stuck with concave, negative-powered glasses, which "de-focus" those parallel rays, and make 'em diverge—just as if they came from a near point.

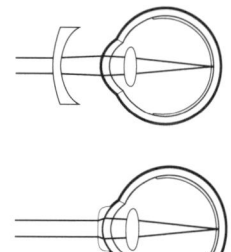

Of course there are also concave contact lenses, which basically create a flatter cornea.

The RK operation truly flattens the cornea, and thus "weakens" the eye and focuses the image on the retina. But let's check out what happens to the nearsighted eye as it enters the presbyopic years.

The Revenge of the Nearsighted

Nearsightedness gets its name from its one advantage—the eye's unwanted excess focal power lets it focus diverging near-point rays easily, without using accommodation. So in middle-aged and senior years, the nearsighted eye can still read easily—you just have to take off your glasses.

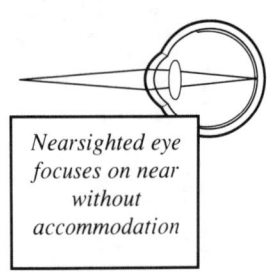

Nearsighted eye focuses on near without accommodation

If you are nearsighted, remove your glasses, close one eye and do the accommodation check we tried a minute ago. The distant background is blurry but your thumb is in focus, without even trying.

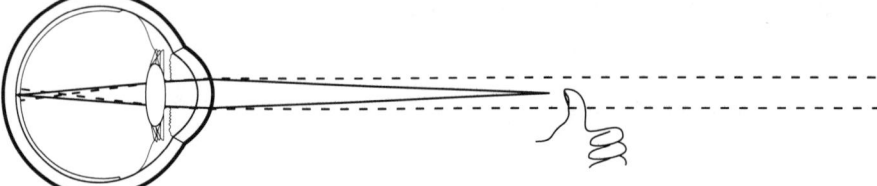

Now put your glasses on. The background becomes clear and your thumb is blurry, until you do some accommodating to focus on it.

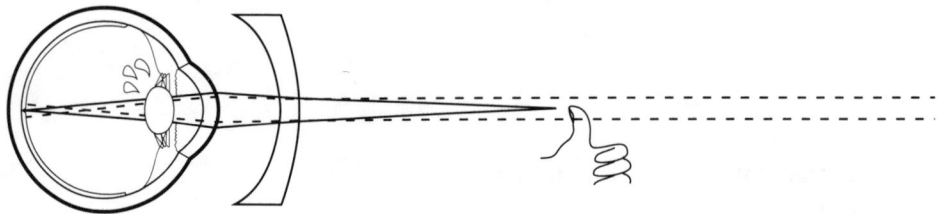

With your glasses or contacts in place, you're in the same boat as the 20/20 eye-owner: you can't read without accommodation, which disappears as you get older.

If you're only slightly nearsighted, you may eventually need bifocals with a weak "plus" segment for reading.

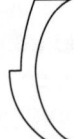

Cross-section of bifocals for very mild myopia: top part is weak minus (concave)lens, lower segment is weak plus (convex) for reading.

On the other hand, if you are too nearsighted to read comfortably without glasses, you'll need bifocals with your regular strong minus-powered distance lens and a weaker minus-powered reading segment.

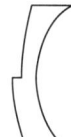

High-myopia bifocals:
Upper part strong minus-powered (concave)
Lower segment, weaker minus

For most nearsighted people, however, reading in later life is just a matter of taking off their glasses.

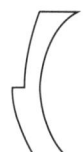

Moderate-myopia bifocals:
Lower segment may have no power (plano)

The One-of-Each Option

Now that contacts are popular—and hard to slip off whenever you want to read—many nearsighted people who reach middle age are opting for "monovision". They wear their distance-correction contact lens in one eye, and leave the other eye nearsighted for reading. For many mildly-nearsighted people, this works fine.

Most people find out about presbyopia when it happens to them, and that's fine since there's nothing they can do about it anyway. If you're contemplating RK you should be aware of it in advance, because if neither eye is nearsighted you'll have to wear glasses to read in your presbyopic years, which hopefully will last for at least three decades. It is better, if possible, to retain some nearsightedness in one eye! Having two different eyes sounds unnatural, but for many people (me included) it works well, with each eye taking over as needed.

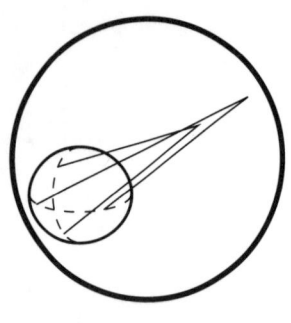

With-the-rule Astigmatism: too strong vertically

The Oval Eye: Astigmatism

With near- and farsightedness it is usually the eye's length that is to blame, although sometimes the cornea is too curved or too flat. Astigmatism is almost always the cornea's fault: instead of being spherical in shape, like a soup spoon, it is slightly elongated and oval, like a teaspoon.

Usually, the cornea is more steeply curved vertically than it is horizontally, like a teaspoon lying on its side. Because the cornea is more curved from top to bottom than from side to side, the eye is more nearsighted vertically than horizontally.

Many nearsighted people have some astigmatism, and it often accompanies farsightedness too—and sometimes it stands alone. Astigmatism can be corrected by making the eyeglass lens slightly cylindrical, so that it adds more power to the flatter axis. Or in the case of the nearsighted person with astigmatism, the concave lens subtracts more power from the steeper axis.

Special contact lenses often work well for astigmatism. And as we'll see, RK can handle mild and moderate astigmatism. Higher degrees require special procedures, and also require you to read Chapter 15.

Units of Eyepower?

Congratulations—you are now the first person on your block to really understand how the eye works and how it changes over time.

Next we'll take a quick look at how vision is measured, so you can read your own prescription and understand it from now on as well as you understand your height and weight. Then on to the fun part.

Optalk: Measuring Refraction

3

When you get a prescription for glasses, the doc tests your eyes in two different ways. There's the subjective eye-chart test: "Read the fifth line from the top and no fair squinting."

But perhaps more important is measuring the actual focal power of your visual optics, just as you might measure the power of a telescope.

The Snellen Visual Acuity Chart

The good old Snellen Chart with the big E on top is the king of the subjective approach. This chart gives us the term 20/20. A doctor in Holland named Snellen had an assistant who was able to read a particular size of type from twenty feet, and the good Dutch doctor thought this man had average vision. Really, that's all 20/20 means—you can read from twenty feet the same line of letters that Snellen's assistant could read from 20 feet.

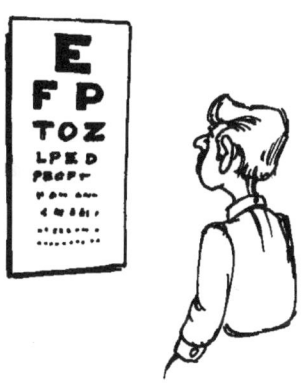

If you can see the smaller line below that one you are beating 20/20, not to mention Snellen's assistant, who would have had to move up to 15 feet to read it. If you can read it at twenty feet, you have 20/15 vision.

Some can even read the tiniest line from 20 feet, the line Snellen's pal could only read from ten feet; they have 20/10. When eye docs gather 'round the campfire, they recount legends of great Sioux warriors even more keen-eyed than that.

If, without glasses, you can barely read the big E on top, that's 20/200: Doc Snellen's assistant could read the big E from 200 feet. But that is still very mild myopia. On the other hand, if you couldn't read the big E even with your glasses on, you would be legally blind.

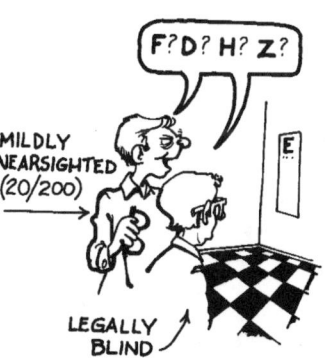

Here's a common variation of the Snellen chart called the E-chart (for some obscure reason.) To use it, put it under a strong light and back up ten feet— size limitations force us to downsize it by 50% and move up from the usual twenty-foot testing distance. It's just for fun anyway. (No fair squinting!)

20/200

20/80

20/40

20/20

20/15

20/10

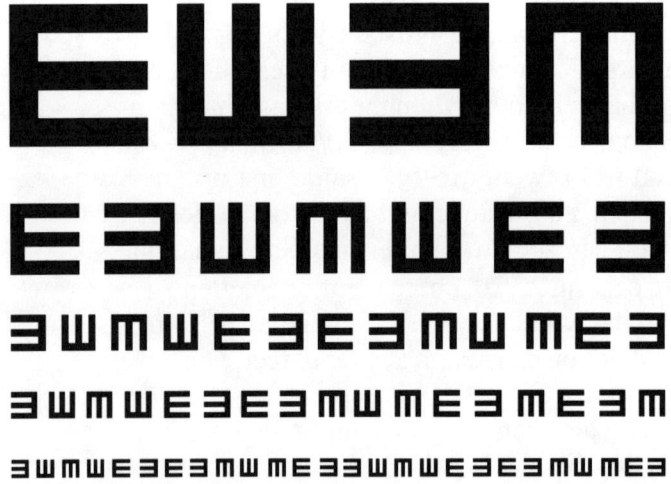

Note: Visual acuity as measured by the Snellen chart is only one part of the complete vision profile now used by many professionals. The profile also includes contrast sensitivity and glare disability, which this chart can't measure.

Meter, Liter, Gram, Diopter

The science of optics has an objective measure for refraction, called the *diopter*. A one-diopter lens focuses light in one meter (about 40 inches).

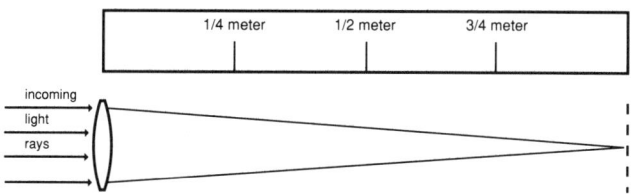

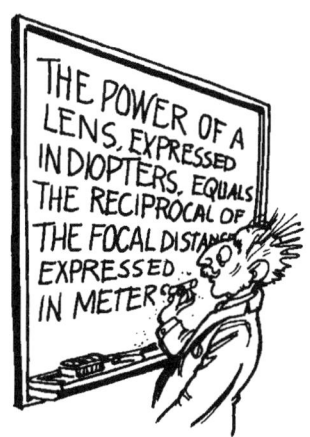

A two-diopter lens would focus in half a meter.

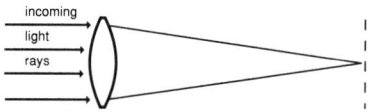

A minus-2-diopter lens (-2 D) will diverge light rays at the same angle as a +2 D lens will focus them.

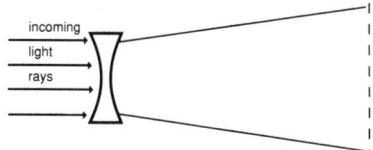

A 4-diopter (4 D) lens will focus light in one fourth of a meter, and so forth. A forty-diopter lens will focus in a fortieth of a meter—about one inch.

The human eye has about sixty diopters: roughly forty-five in the cornea and fifteen in the lens. So it can focus in one sixtieth of a meter, or two-thirds of an inch, which in fact is how much focusing room you have between your lens and your retina.

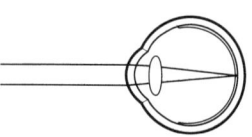

Most nearsighted people's eyes are too strong by just a few diopters. There is only a rough correlation between diopters and eye-chart acuity, but a person who is within one diopter of "emmetropia", or perfect focus, is usually 20/40 or better. Most people with vision in that range can do without glasses most or all of the time.

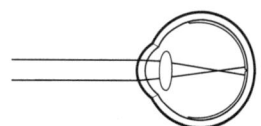

Refraction and Prescription

Your "refraction" in op-talk is the objective measure of your eye's focal power, while your lens prescription tells the optician what power of lenses the optometrist or ophthalmologist thinks you should have. Usually they are the same.

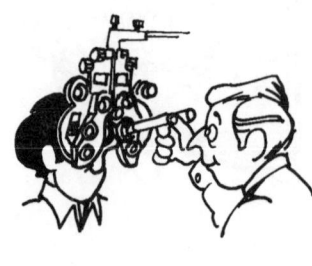

The eye professional who "takes your refraction"—either an optometrist ("well-eye doctor") or an ophthalmologist (eye-specializing M.D.)—will use several ingenious optical gadgets to obtain an objective measurement of your vision. To make sure you aren't involuntarily accommodating and thereby increasing your focal power, eyedrops may be applied to relax your lens' little muscle.

Do you know what your refraction is? Few people do! Find out—either call your eye professional, or just drop by an optician's shop and have them measure your glasses.

A typical nearsightedness refraction looks something like this:

O.D. -3.50
O.S. -3.00

That "O.D." stands for oculis dexter, or right eye. O.S. stands for Oculis Sinister, which sounds like a science-fiction villain, doesn't it? Means left eye, of course. (If both eyes are the same it might say O.U., meaning Both Eyes.) The minus sign is used because the myopic eye is corrected with a negative-powered, concave lens, which subtracts focusing power from the too-strong eye.

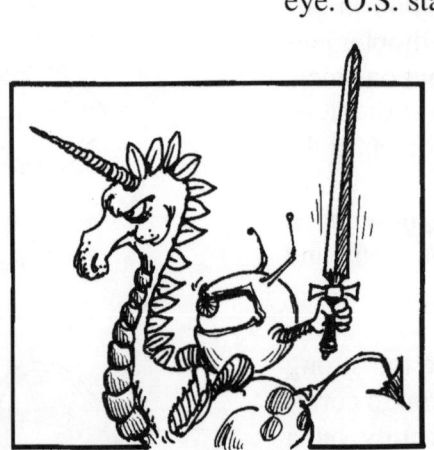

Oculis Sinister, Warlord of Opia

This person has three and a half diopters of nearsight in the right eye and three in the left, so in conversational terms he or she would be called "a three-diopter myope", or "a person with 3 D of nearsightedness", or "a minus-three".

No Stigma

If you have astigmatism there will be two more numbers. The first tells how much of it you have—how much more curved the cornea is in one axis than another. The second number tells the axis of the cylindrical component of your eyeglasses. For example: O.D.-3.50 -1.00 x 180.

This is a prescription for astigmatism of one diopter, at the 180-degree ("with-the-rule") axis. If that last number is 180 or close, then you have with-the-rule astigmatism; if it's 90 or thereabouts you have against-the rule astigmatism.

Just to confuse us further, the professionals use two different forms of describing astigmatic errors. The above is "minus form", as you can tell by the minus sign in front of the one. Ask to have your prescription written in minus form, which we'll use in this book. (See Chapter 15 for more on this.)

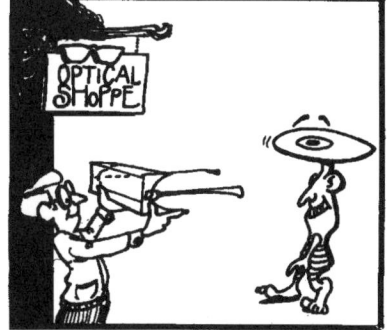

Cylindrical lens for with-the-rule astigmatism. The axis of the lens is horizontal (180); the extra power is vertical (90)

Now You're Reading Eyenglish

Here are a few more examples:

-7.00 -.50 x 90 (a seven-diopter "high myope" with half a diopter of against-the-rule astigmatism).

-2.00 -1.00 x 180 (two mild diopters of nearsightedness with one diopter of with-the-rule astigmatism).

Farsightedness is shown with a plus sign: for example, O.D. +3.50. It takes a positive (plus) lens to add the focusing power that is missing in a farsighted eye—that is, a convex lens like a magnifying glass.

Once you're in the presbyopic years, there will probably be another part to your prescription, an "add" for bifocals. "Add 1.50 D" would be typical.

Next, let's talk about nearsightedness for a few minutes, and then we'll get into the RK operation.

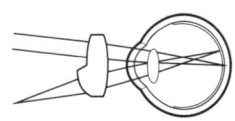

Bifocals

Hey Strong-Eyes! 4

Nearsightedness is Too Much of a Good Thing

Nearsighted people don't have "weak eyes", but just the opposite: our eyes have too much focusing power.

Normally, when a writer is discussing some handicap or problem, he starts with a list of famous people who succeeded in spite of it. With myopia, it would almost be harder to produce a list of great men and women who succeeded without it.

Mount Rushmore Wears Glasses

I'll just mention my favorite President, Teddy Roosevelt. Courageous, brilliant, creative, energetic: Teddy was the classic nearsighted character. He had health problems as a child, but he doggedly overcame them and I'll bet T.R. would have taken a keen interest in Radial Keratotomy.

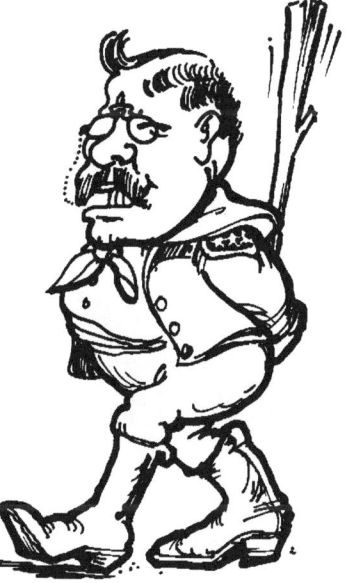

Of course you don't have to be nearsighted to be President, but there is no question that a disproportionate number of super-achievers and great thinkers are nearsighted. As I researched this book I actually started to be slightly prejudiced against non-myopes (a lazy, sluggish buncha cold fish they are) and very bitter about anti-myope hiring rules, which cost our police and fire departments dearly in lost talent.

Is Myopia Preventable?

There has been plenty of debate over the causes of nearsightedness. The long-standing assumption that it is hereditary has never been proven, and may be untrue. The great question is: does childhood reading cause nearsightedness?

The connection has long been suspected because nearsighted children are so often bookworms and because myopia, rare a few generations ago, has undergone an explosion to become the most common visual problem in literate countries. Dr. Francis Young of Washington State University has convincingly shown a connection: in one famous study, he showed that the first generations of Alaskan Eskimos to be taught reading in childhood experienced an exponential increase in myopia compared to their parents and grandparents.

For Some Kids, Maybe

Dr. Young, probably the world's foremost researcher into the causes of myopia, believes that the constant accommodation of reading or other close work—including television viewing—causes the youthful eye to elongate. A child's glasses aggravate the problem by increasing the amount of accommodation needed for reading. He feels that if it were not for glasses, few children would become more than mildly myopic because, as we've seen, mild myopia allows effortless reading without accommodation. But when a nearsighted child wears his glasses while reading, he must accommodate as much as a 20/20 child. The renewed accommodation may cause increased myopia, requiring a new, stronger prescription, causing more myopia, and so on: a vicious circle.

Why would accommodation make the eye elongate? Perhaps because there is a feedback mechanism that normally keeps the eye in proper focus as it grows, keeping the curvature of the cornea and the length of the eye in proportion. Suppose the eye was too short, and therefore too weak (farsighted). This would result in excessive accommodating, which would send a signal: *We're working too hard, we need more focal power.* The feedback system would respond by

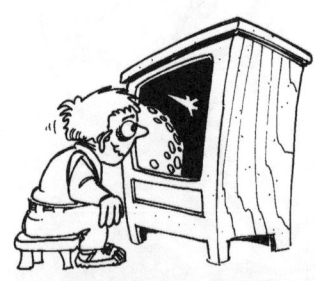

There's strong evidence that nearsightedness is dramatically increasing due to children watching TV from a few feet away. Make the kids sit at least ten feet back!

lengthening the eye a bit, giving more room for the image to focus—which normally would relieve the need for so much accommodating. This mechanism would guarantee a reasonably well-focused eye. Perhaps reading, by requiring constant accommodation, "tricks" the system, and makes the eye keep elongating even though it isn't farsighted.

I'd rather be nearsighted than have missed out on any childhood reading and book-larnin', but maybe we should teach the kids to give their eyes a break more often when they read, and if they are already nearsighted, to take off their glasses for reading. If they do that they won't have to accommodate, and the vicious circle will be broken. Some experts, including Dr. Young, feel that by giving every child plus-powered reading glasses when he first starts to read, myopia could be entirely prevented.

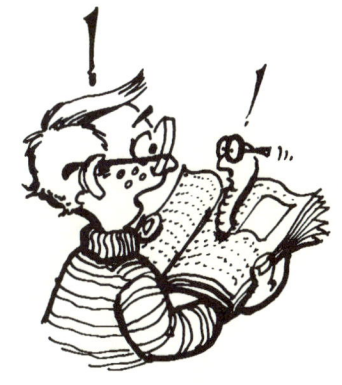

For more information on this and other approaches to preventing myopia, contact the Optometric Extension Program Foundation, Inc., 2912 South Daimler, Santa Ana California 92705 (714-250-8070)

Myopia Versus Barbarism?

Our negative feelings toward nearsightedness are skewed by the fact that with today's availability of reading glasses, we don't need it any more. To be fair we should remember that nearsightedness prevents the loss of near vision in middle age, and that until a few centuries ago only nearsighted men and women could see close work past the age of fifty. Even though the average lifespan was short in primitive times, there were always some who did reach old age, and they were often the very people who specialized in close work—weavers, net-makers, tool-makers and arrowsmiths.

Suppose the young apprentice arrowsmith or needleworker became nearsighted due to many hours of intense accommodation—this meant he or she would have terrible distance vision, and never be a hunter or raider, but would be able to see close work closer than others, and more impor-

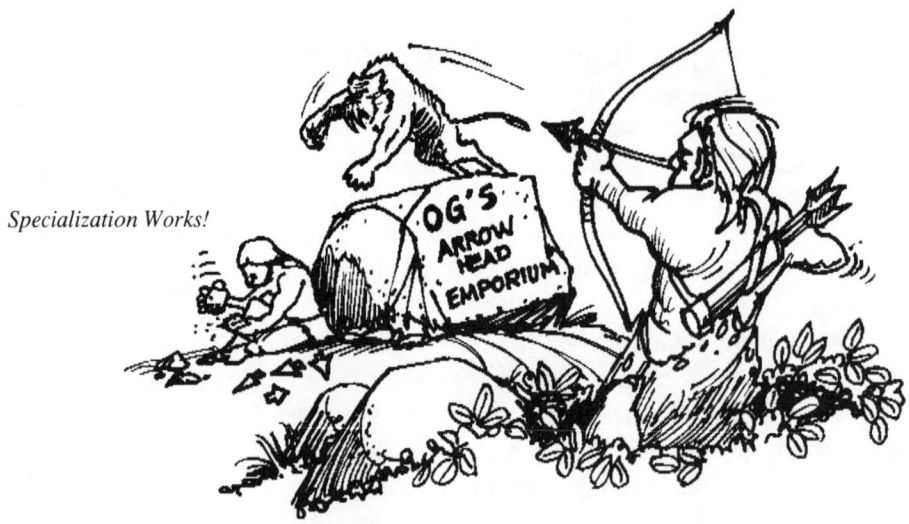

Specialization Works!

tantly would be able to keep on seeing close work in old age, to the benefit of the entire tribe.

Nearsightedness is a positive word; it speaks of what must have been a real blessing in the days before glasses. Probably it gave a boost to the development of writing, since it enabled scholarly types to go on working with letters clear through their lives. In fact, it may be that myopia promoted many kinds of specialization and hastened the dawn of civilization.

Just the same, modern civilization has certainly led to an excessive amount of nearsightedness, and we definitely don't need it now. Hopefully we will learn to prevent as well as cure it.

Natural, Holistic, Wholesome, and Questionable

You may have heard of the "Bates Method" and its modern disciples. These enthusiasts of holistic medicine, an approach toward health that often has important things to say, believe that nearly all visual problems can be solved by the right ideas, attitude, and exercises.

According to these folks, the nearsighted eye is unhealthy and reflects mind/body imbalance. Sci-

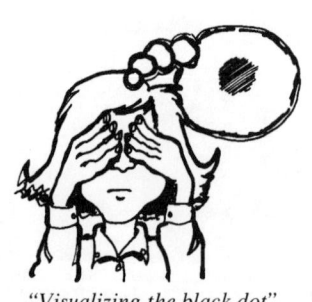

"Visualizing the black dot" is one Bates technique.

entific medicine has problems with that because in fact most visual errors are caused by simple variations in the proportionate sizes and curvatures of various parts of the eye.

Probably the only type of myopia that may be under the nearsighted adult's control is a phenomenon called "pseudo-myopia", in which the eye accommodates needlessly, making you even more nearsighted than you are to begin with.

Pseudo-myopia (also called "school myopia") can be detected only by an eye doctor doing a "cycloplegic refraction", testing your eyes after administering eyedrops which shut down the involuntary accommodation. If you learn that part of your myopia is pseudo-myopia, possibly the Bates Method will help you to relax your accommodation and eliminate this problem.

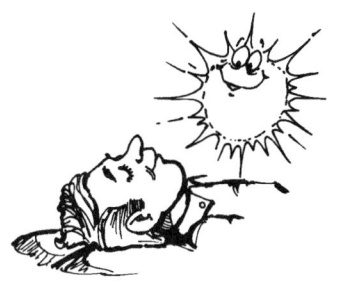

"Sunning" - another Bates technique.

It's possible that some people can train the muscle that controls the lens so well that they can even correct some of their true myopia. A biofeedback device called the "Accommotrac" has been developed to help in this attempt; it emits a tone that tells you when your focus is improving. Supposedly some patients have licked their nearsightedness in the course of twenty or more one-hour sessions. If you're interested, call around and you may find an optometrist or ophthalmologist in your area who has this machine.

The Mash-It-Flat Approach

Another approach is called Orthokeratology, which consists of flattening the cornea by wearing tight-fitting hard contact lenses. Each successive pair of lenses is flatter than the last pair, and gradually the cornea is "trained" to lie flat enough to provide improved vision. Supposedly, if successful, the patient will eventually only need to wear the training lenses occasionally, to keep his corneas from returning to their original shape. Most ophthalmologists feel that this is a bad way to treat a cornea, since it forces living tissue into an unnatural shape and impedes the cornea's oxygen supply in the process. The results are often unpredictable or impermanent—in fact, many RK patients have been unhappy orthokeratology alumni who have seen the effect of cornea-flattening but want a more permanent result.

The Time-Honored Nuisances

Until the past few centuries the only help for nearsightedness was squinting or using a pinhole—in fact the word "myopia" means squint-vision. Many kids still use these methods until they are dragged kicking and screaming to the optician.

Glasses are the most time-honored solution to myopia. The concave lens, which "de-focuses" light in order to counteract the myopic eye's excess focus, was probably invented much more recently than the plus-powered, convex lens for farsightedness and presbyopic near-vision. After all, the convex lens is easier to make, and occurs more often in nature (icicles, gemstones, beads, water droplets etc.). Also, myopia was quite rare until the last few generations, while presbyopia has been around forever.

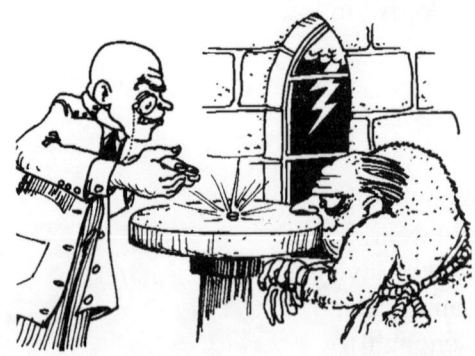

The contact lens, invented by the heinous Baron von Contact (Editor's note: Horsefeathers. See Appendix B) first became popular in the fifties, but caused so many disasters that it remained controversial until the soft version was invented in 1966. It is now used by about 20 million Americans, and provides more natural, undistorted vision with less impact on appearance than glasses. Rather than get into contact lenses here, we've put a whole appendix on them in the back of the book.

My Opia is Stronger Than Yours Is, So There

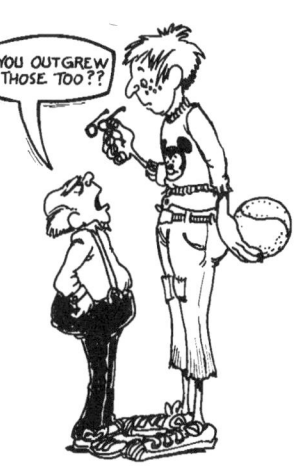

Most myopia first becomes apparent at the age of eight or ten, and is discovered at school. It slowly increases as the child grows, and sometimes correlates to periods of intense schoolwork or TV-watching. Nearsightedness usually stabilizes about when height does, around age 18 or 20.

Degrees of myopia vary greatly. One person may have a diopter and a half too much focusing power (-1.50 D), and be able to see clearly out to thirty inches. Another will have six diopters of myopia (-6 D), and see clearly only within a seven-inch range. Even the mildly-nearsighted among us are likely to be "legally blind without glasses", so don't ever let that phrase scare you.

Low degrees are more common, with increasingly high myopia increasingly rare. Vision forms a bell-shaped curve on a graph, with no truly "normal" or "abnormal" level.

How myopic are you? Hopefully, you have your prescription or "refraction" in hand. An easy way to get a rough idea is to have an optician measure your current glasses. Even rougher: check the following guide.

Myopia Rough Test (for Funsies)

Test one eye at a time, without glasses. Hold the book out where it's blurry and bring it closer until you can read the letters. Whatever fraction of a meter (forty inches) you can read at will tell you how many surplus diopters you've got (your refraction) and how many negative ones you'll need in your glasses (your prescription). For example, if you can focus on letters half a meter away (20 inches), you have 2 diopters of myopia (-2 D); if you can only focus 1/4 meter away (10 inches) that's four diopters of myopia (-4 D).

Knowing the diopters doesn't tell you the Snellen-chart acuity. There are some other major variables to complicate the picture, starting with astigmatism. Also, no cornea is quite spherical—fortunately, since spherical lenses have a problem called spherical aberration, which would detract from sharp vision. Optically, the cornea has a certain mystique. But this little self-test will give you a rough idea of how nearsighted you are. (Warning: if you have astigmatism as well as myopia, it won't work too well.)

Here Goes:

If you can barely read the page (without glasses) at:

40 inches (about one meter): that's -1.00 D. With this you will probably have 20/40 vision, good enough to drive legally in most states.

26 inches: that's -1.50 D or 1.5 diopters of nearsightedness.

20 inches: that's -2.00 D. Might have 20/200.

13 inches: -3.00. Some of the nicest people have this prescription. [Editor's note: this was the author's prescription]

11 inches: -3.50, moderate myopia.

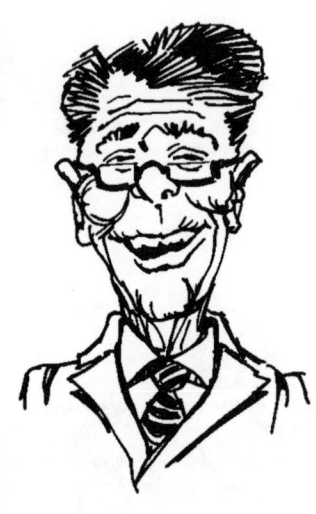

9 inches: -4.00, four diopters. Ronald Reagan's prescription, and it gave him hell in his early acting career, before he adjusted to contacts. As President, he wore one contact for distance and kept the other eye nearsighted for reading.

6 inches: -6.50. This is getting into high myopia. Can hardly find way around house without glasses. Unless you're over forty, this is as much nearsightedness as RK can generally handle.

4 inches: -10.00 D. Truly handicapped without glasses; "count-fingers" vision at two feet.

Less than 4 inches: more than ten diopters of myopia. This is "very high" myopia. There are several stronger-than-RK alternatives; see Ch.14.

A Nice Test to Score Low On

Low myopia—below three diopters—is usually a fairly minor inconvenience. Unfortunately, probably unfairly, it keeps people out of some exciting professions: police work, firefighting, paramedical, piloting. For other jobs it's an inconvenience, if not an absolute obstacle.

Low myopia can also complicate many sports—swimming, diving, surfing, skiing. And if you must wear glasses, it has an impact on your appearance which you may or may not appreciate. But glasses for low myopia don't cause much distortion, because they don't have to be very thick. And several types of contact lenses are available—daily-wear soft lenses, the more hazardous extended-wear lenses, new gas-permeable rigid lenses, and now even disposable ones.

Also, as we will see, RK is most likely to be a complete success for low myopia.

One 'Opia Versus the Other

Low myopia is great "presbyopia insurance", because it only takes about two and a half diopters of myopia to make up for the accommodation ability of the lens that is lost by age 65. So as we've mentioned, the -2 D or -3 D myope usually reads without glasses in senior years. If he's a contact wearer, he may be like Ronald Reagan and wear just one contact lens at a time (usually in the dominant eye) and leave the other eye's myopia as built-in reading glasses.

The presbyopic -1D "mini-myope" will probably wear bifocals, with a weak plus segment for reading and a weak minus lens for distance, or may wear two different-powered contacts. (Although for interesting optical reasons, the presbyopic glasses-wearing myope has considerably greater easy-vision range than he has with contacts, or a non-myope would have.)

Moderation in All Things?

Moderate myopia, from three to six diopters, is considerably more of a nuisance. A -5 D myope has to wear glasses to read, or else hold the book within seven inches of his face. While the low myope can function well enough without glasses for swimming or using a public shower (or finding misplaced glasses), these things can be a hassle for the moderate myope.

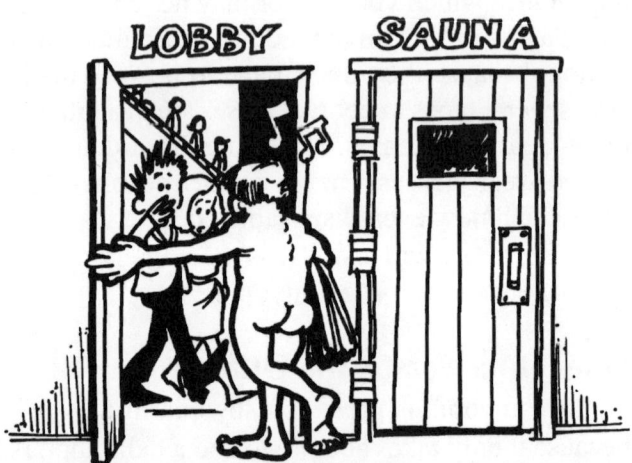

Glasses for this degree of myopia are a little thicker, heavier, and cause some distortion and shrinkage of the visual field. Contact lenses are also a little thicker.

As presbyopia sets in, the moderate nearsightee will probably wear bifocals with his lifelong distance correction and a weaker segment for near, weak enough to leave sufficient surplus power for reading.

For the moderately nearsighted person, RK still offers perhaps a 75%-or-better chance of escaping glasses—which may be good enough for those who strongly dislike eyewear. We'll examine these odds more closely in another chapter.

The Samson of Eyes

High myopia—generally greater than six diopters, and sometimes as high as twenty or more—can be devilish. These eyes are much too strong, usually because they are too long, and their error can't be easily corrected with glasses. You get "barrel-distortion": things bulge in the middle; squares appear barrel-shaped. The size of the image is reduced, and the field is decreased. Peripheral vision is history.

The highly myopic eye also may have poor contrast sensitivity—that is, although with glasses on you may do fine with the black-and-white Snellen chart, in the real world of shades-of-grey you may have trouble making out subtle contrasts. Myopes also often suffer from "glare disability", which means that glare from headlights at night, or bright sunshine, can be troublesome. Only recently have methods been devised for testing these important functions, which along with visual acuity (a la Snellen) are used to compile your complete vision profile.

Unless you can handle contacts (and high-myopia contacts are thicker and more uncomfortable than others) high myopia can restrict your lifestyle, and it can even be dangerous in emergencies. Highly myopic people have been a driving force for refractive surgery, badgering ophthalmologists, cuffing their ears and voluteering for new procedures.

You Tough Cases get Extra Chapters for the Same Price! Such a Deal

High myopia and astigmatism complicate the RK picture, so we have special chapters on both of them. RK rarely corrects more than six or seven diopters in younger patients (under 40); for some older patients it can correct up to twelve diopters. But there are several other options that we'll discuss. The highly astigmatic person can be helped by "Astigmatic Keratotomy", or AK, a rapidly developing area of ophthalmology.

Before we leave the general subject of being nearsighted, it's fair to note that the Scouts' Rule applies: Be Prepared with your best corrected vision. Whether you use glasses, contacts, RK or whatever, be equipped with good sight. Don't go around blurry-sighted; this world is too beautiful and too dangerous for that.

Now let's take a look at the way Radial Keratotomy works to correct myopia.

How RK Does It   5

The idea of correcting myopia by flattening the cornea, and thereby decreasing its excessive focalpower, has been around for a long time. The first surgeon to try it was a Japanese ophthalmologist, Dr. Sato, who operated on a series of patients before and after World War Two. Unfortunately, he made big mistakes (such as operating on the inner side of the cornea), and although the surgery was effective it caused corneal clouding years later, so the whole idea was discredited for a time.

The Punch Heard 'round the World

In the early seventies, according to legend, the Russian eye surgeon Svyatislav Fyodorov examined a nearsighted teenager who had been punched in the eye in a fistfight, and whose cornea had been radially scratched by his broken glasses. Astonishingly, the eye was no longer nearsighted. Professor Fyodorov decided that if a schoolyard bully could correct nearsightedness, an ophthalmologist should also be able to. He and his associates spent several years developing an operation that used tiny radial incisions to flatten the cornea.

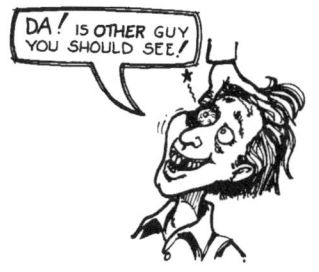

Fyodorov's results were encouraging, and several energetic American surgeons led by Dr. Leo Bores of Scottsdale, Arizona, picked up the ball. They gave the operation the name Radial Keratotomy, or RK, and introduced it to the U.S. in 1978. A team at the University of Southern California led by Dr. James J. Salz and Dr. Richard Villasenor investigated the operation scientifically and figured out how it really worked, which led to important changes—it was found that fewer and smaller incisions could be used, making the operation safer and the recovery less painful. A safer,

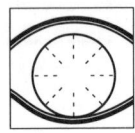

RK, actual size. Incisions are invisible soon after operation.

more reliable technique, called the "American technique", was developed. Many surgeons made important contributions, and much better instruments were developed. RK became very much an American phenomenon, with thousands of Americans having the operation every month.

PERKing Right Along

In 1981 the National Eye Institute backed an impressive study of 435 patients called the Prospective Examination of Radial Keratotomy, or "PERK Study", which followed the patients from their pre-operative exam through surgery and for five years afterward. RK was found to be reasonably safe and effective, although not perfectly predictable. The new alternative was on its way, although not without controversy, as we'll see.

Radial Keratotomy means "radial cornea incision". In most types of surgery, you make an incision in order to do something on the other side of it, but in RK getting there is *all* the fun. The whole ballgame consists of making tiny cuts in the cornea about an eighth of an inch long and a fiftieth of an inch deep—not even all the way through the cornea. No other part of the eye is involved, nothing is removed or installed, there are no stitches or injections required. It's a very little surgery that goes a long way, thanks to the cornea being the curious little critter that it is.

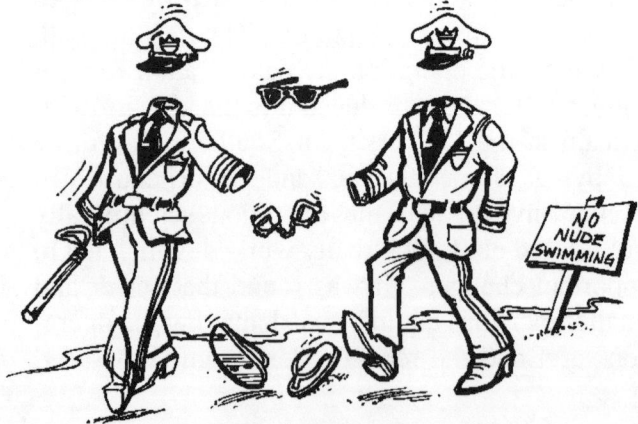

If your whole body was built like the cornea

"No, Johnny, That's Cornwall!"

The cornea is not where Cornish hens come from, as the schoolboy thought. It's that most beautiful and special part of the body's surface, our built-in jewel, our window on the world: so transparent that it can't actually be seen at all, only reflections off of the tear film that covers it. The cornea is the "invisible man" in all of us.

Close one eye and press a finger against the eyelid, and move your eyes from side to side. You can feel the little rounded bulge of the cornea moving back and forth. It's firm, pressurized, yet slightly flexible. It isn't jelly-like or disgusting. It's wonderful, ingenious, healthy and strong.

In fact, the cornea is a surprisingly tough little customer, with three main layers of cell tissues, and two thin membranes sandwiched between them.

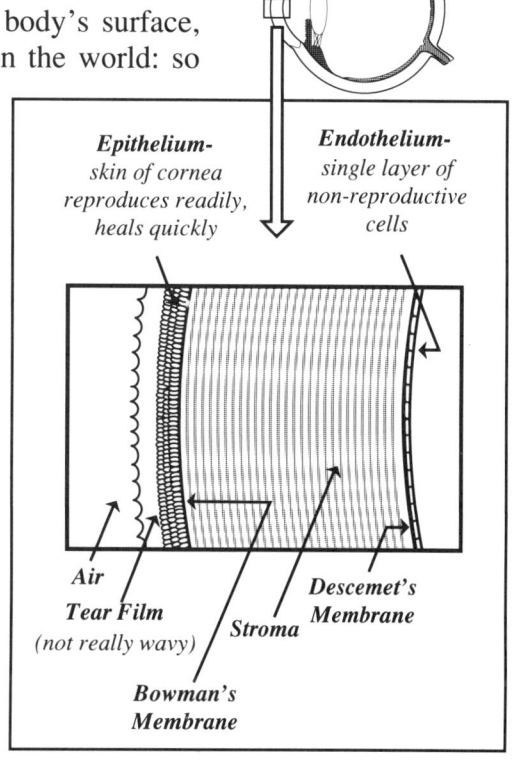

Well Bless Your Leathery Hide

The first layer, exposed to the hazards of our dangerous planet, is a thin sheet of actual skin. Like all skin, its cells are constantly sloughing off at the surface as new cells are born underneath—in fact, these cells live only seven days before they are washed away by the tear film. This *epithelium*

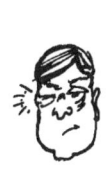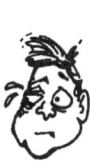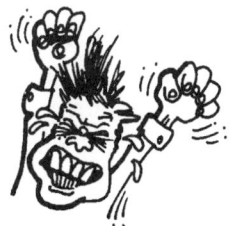

Author experiencing foreign-body sensation (2-second-interval photographs)

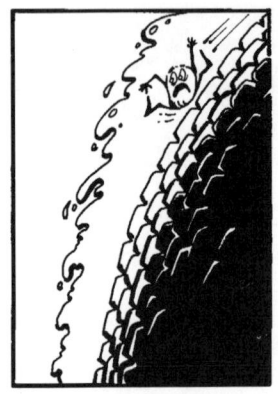

Epithelial cell getting sloughed

is about five cell-layers thick, and it is bristling with tiny nerve endings—more of them than any other surface of the body, and every one just dying to scream bloody murder and trigger some kind of response at the least provocation.

What a merry short life the epithelial cells lead. They can reproduce at a dizzying rate, which is why the cornea can heal in a few hours after you remove a scratchy particle from your eye. This fast regrowth is important to RK, because the epithelium quickly grows over the incisions, plugs them up and seals them off from outside sources of infection.

Oh Baby, You Sure Are Built!

Below the epithelium lies the microscopically-thin *Bowman's Membrane*, which gives the epithelium something to hold onto. Below it lies the main body of the cornea, the *Stroma*. This thick layer is itself composed of about 250 layers of connective tissue, the same kind of tough, stringy tissue that your ligaments are made of. These tough fibers are produced by cells, and those cells are still in there somewhere, hiding. But they don't seem to reproduce much (in fact they don't seem to have any fun at all) so this part of the cornea can take a long time to heal.

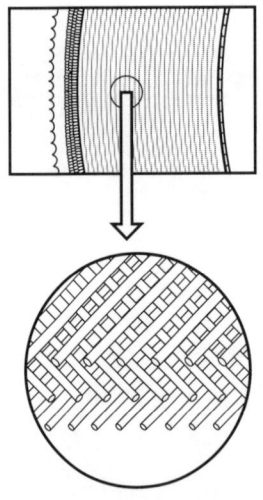

Stroma
50 Layers of connective tissue laid at right angles to each other

Where Angels Fear to Tread, Let Alone Ophthalmologists

The innermost layer of the cornea is a very thin skin called the *endothelium,* which consists of one single layer of cells. This fragile inner skin of the cornea should not be disturbed, and leaving it alone is a major goal of any eye operation. You could say that the endothelium is to eye surgeons what Social Security is to politicians.

So that's the cornea, the watchglass of the eye: basically, a thick layer of tough connective tissue, with a robust skin protecting it from the great outdoors and a delicate membrane sealing it off from the interior of the eye. It is thinnest in the center—a little more than half a millimeter thick—and about 30% thicker toward the outer edge.

It's Not Just for Decoration, Either

The cornea is strongly curved and has a lot of focusing power—about 45 diopters, roughly 80% of the eye's total focusing strength. (If you've ever opened your eyes underwater, you know what the world would look like if the cornea lost its power!) If your cornea is just 5% too strongly curved, giving you an extra 2 diopters, you probably can't read the big E on the Snellen chart. So you can see that just a small amount of flattening would be required to correct moderate nearsightedness.

Although the whole cornea is transparent, the most important part of it is the optical zone. This is the central area, over the pupil—whatever it is you are looking at is seen through here. The visual axis, an imaginary line between whatever you are staring at and the retina's hyper-receptive central area, passes through the center of the cornea's central optical zone. This is the part of the cornea where a good focus really matters. The outer, or peripheral, cornea is much less important.

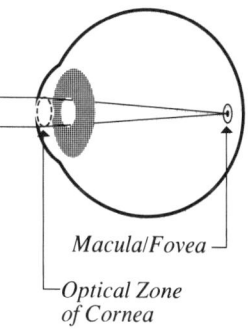

Macula/Fovea

Optical Zone of Cornea

Make It Right, Doc, But Don't Touch it

So the goal of RK is to flatten this small central area, without touching it. No incisions can be made here, because the tiny scars could cause diffusion of the light on its way to the fovea, and interfere with the precise central vision we demand. This little central circle over the pupil, about 3mm in diameter, is both the target and the forbidden zone of RK.

The RK operation consists of a number of "relaxing incisions", which start just outside of the central optical zone and radiate out toward the perimeter of the cornea, where it fastens to the white of the eye. The incisions are about an eighth of an inch long, and about as deep as three sheets of this paper, so the total amount of cutting involved is minute. But as they say, minor surgery is what the other fellow has. And in fact from the cornea's point of view four or eight cuts that go 90% through it is pretty major.

Why It Works

The incisions temporarily weaken the peripheral cornea, which immediately bulges outward slightly due to the pressure of the aqueous fluid inside the eye (intraocular pressure). And as the peripheral cornea bulges outward, the central zone flattens inward. Because it flattens, its focusing power decreases—the too-strong myopic eye is made a little less strong.

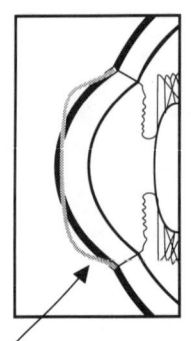

Grey line represents shape of cornea after RK, horrendously exaggerated

The more incisions that are made, the deeper the incisions are cut, and the closer in toward the center the incisions are extended, the more the cornea bulges outward in the periphery and flattens in the center. So these are the three variables by which the effect of the operation is determined.

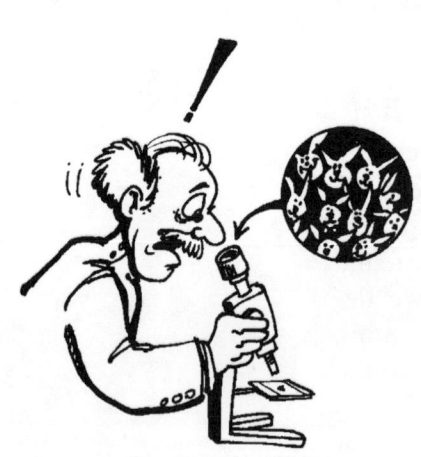

After the surgery, the outer epithelium heals very quickly—its prolific cells reproducing like rabbits can only dream of—and plugs the incisions at the surface. The thicker stroma layer grows back into the incisions in the weeks and months, even years, that follow, and as it heals the cornea solidifies in its new flatter shape. The eye's optical properties are permanently changed.

The body tries to heal itself in its original shape as much as possible, so the cornea may regress slightly toward its pre-RK shape as it heals. In older patients it doesn't try as hard, so RK is more effective in your forties or fifties than it is when you're a mere lad of thirty-five like me. As we'll see, in some cases the cornea continues to flatten slightly for several years.

There's No Stopping Us Now

We are really covering ground! First we laid the foundation for a true understanding of refractive surgery, RK in particular. Now we've examined the invisible—your cornea—and we've seen how RK changes your optics. Next we'll run through the eye examination, and then we'll look at the fantastic choices involved in the planning of your operation.

You Can't Cram for a Pre-RK Exam   6

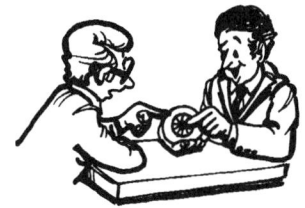

Before you can have the RK operation, or even make an informed decision on whether to go ahead with it, you have to find a qualified surgeon and present yourself for a complete eye examination. It also helps if you can determine whether you will want one eye corrected or both, and you and your doctor have some other planning to do. Chapter 16 will help with choosing a surgeon, and the next couple of chapters will discuss monovision and the planning process. First, the RK Exam.

The $75 or thereabouts that this exam will cost is money well spent. Everybody should have their eyes inspected every few years, if only to check for sneaky diseases such as glaucoma, the silent, symptomless stealer of sight. If diagnosed early this common disease can be arrested and completely controlled, but if you wait until you notice that your vision is failing it will probably be too late to undo the damage.

Don't be a Stranger

In addition to eye diseases, wider problems like hypertension and diabetes often can be diagnosed in an eye examination. And all sorts of minor nuisances can be discovered and fixed by an ophthalmologist—things like eyelid inflammations and styes, ingrown eyelashes, a "lazy eye", or an obsolete eyewear prescription. Every eye-owner ought to darken his ophthalmologist's door every couple of years, even if not considering RK.

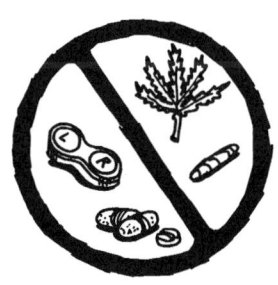

It's very important that you not wear soft contact lenses, or use any prescription (or recreational) drugs, for at least two weeks prior to a pre-

RK exam, unless you clear it with the doctor. Hard contacts should not be worn for at least a month before the exam.

The doctor will ask your medical history. Medical histories vary, like those of nations; don't be ashamed if yours is as stormy as Ireland's. Be sure to mention if you or any close relative has had any problems with crossed or "lazy" eyes, even in early childhood. The doctor will also want to know what drugs you may use.

Cheech and Chong Might Have a Problem with RK

Mention any prescription drugs you are taking, and illegal ones too. The ophthalmologist won't get excited and call your mother if you say you smoke marijuana; the fact is that perhaps a quarter of people in the usual RK age range use pot. Marijuana can play havoc with the effect of RK because it sometimes lowers the pressure inside the eye—lowers it a lot, possibly to half what it should be—and this detracts from the effect of the operation, which depends on that "intraocular pressure" to hold the cornea in its new shape. Anyone considering RK should stop using pot at least two weeks before the examination, and not use it at all during the recovery period. (For that matter, the fact that pot can have such weird and unexplained effects might make you think about not resuming the habit at all.)

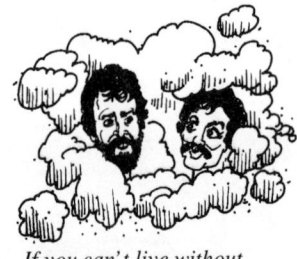

*If you can't live without marijuana, you'd better resolve **that** problem before you have RK!*

Eyeing and Snellen

The doc will test your vision. First, your visual acuity: the good old Snellen Eye Chart. Which is the smallest line of print you can read? You'll be tested for unaided vision, as well as with your glasses.

Then, the doc will "take your refraction". This is a more objective test of how strong your focus is—how many diopters nearsighted or farsighted you are. For this, the doctor will use the phoropter, the butterfly-shaped device with about a billion lens combinations in it, and a little flashlight called a retinoscope. You'll be asked to judge "which is better: number one or number two?" repeatedly, while the doc tries various corrections, until he or she is certain of your refraction, including the axis of your astigmatism if you have any.

This test is usually done a second time after eyedrops are administered which relax the lens muscles. Some nearsighted people involuntarily accommodate, making them even more nearsighted—a phenomenon called "pseudomyopia". So the ophthalmologist will give you cycloplegic eyedrops to paralyze your lens muscle, to make sure he doesn't overdo the RK and correct more myopia than you really have.

Boyoboy, do those drops sting! This is the most painful second of the whole RK experience.

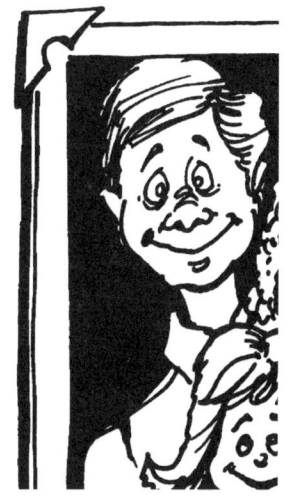

A Necessary Eyeful

Something else about cycloplegic eyedrops: they relax another muscle to an even more comatose state than the muscle that works the lens. What really gets zonked is the muscle that closes your iris—the drops make your iris open amazingly wide and stay that way for about 24 or 36 hours, obliging you to wear sunglasses outdoors, so have a pair handy. Your pupils will look enormous; don't plan on having any family pictures taken right after the eye exam unless you want to scare your relatives.

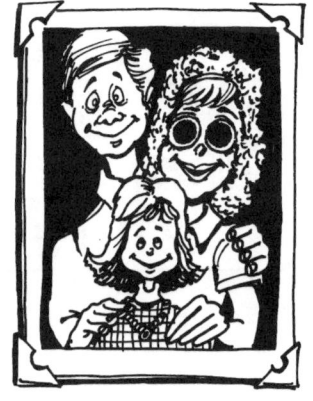

In spite of its annoyance, the "cycloplegic refraction" is a necessary part of the pre-RK exam. Cycloplegia also provides a good opportunity to preview presbyopia: like complete presbyopia, it leaves you with no accommodation, no ability to focus on near objects. Observe that with your glasses on, you cannot read—just as the 20/20 eye can't read unaided in post-40 years. Without glasses, your nearsighted eye can still see close up—its surplus focusing power does the trick. This fact is worth appreciating.

The doc will proceed to check a lot of little things. Any eyelid inflammations or disorders? How's that big blue (brown, green, grey) iris doing? The doc will check your "rotations": are your eyes still working together well? And your visual fields: do you still have that ambush-proof peripheral vision?

So Lay Your Head Upon My Slit-lamp

Then he'll set your chin in a slit-lamp microscope and look inside those little round movie theaters. Corneas nice and clean, no scars or thin spots? Lenses in good shape, no incipient cataracts starting to cloud them up?

While the doc has your face conveniently immobilized, he'll produce a little guage called a tonometer and by touching it to the surface of your cornea, quickly measure the pressure of the liquid interior of your eye—which, like air in a tire, allows the eye to hold its shape. Abnormally high pressure could mean glaucoma, a potential tragedy which can be prevented or greatly lessened if it is discovered early. Sadly, there are no apparent symptoms of chronic glaucoma that the patient can observe before it's too late. The excessive pressure slowly cuts off the blood supply to the optic nerve, but by the time you notice the narrowing of your vision, it may be too late to prevent permanent damage. So as you get older, get wiser too, and see your ophthalmologist more often!

As far as RK is concerned, however, low pressure is more likely to be a problem than high pressure. The pressure inside the eye is what forces the cornea into its new, flatter shape.

How Are You 137 Million Guys Doing In There?

Now to explore the crystalline depths. The doc gets out the ophthalmoscope and peers through its light beam for a magnified view of your retina, at the very back of the eye. The retina is like a small, brave colony of brain cells. Here, in plain view, are nerves, nerve fibers and blood vessels, the living wires and pipes of the human machine. The eye is our window on the world, and by the same token a window on ourselves. Several diseases can be spotted here before they make themselves known in any other way. Also, the retinal tears, detachments and other problems that sometimes happen to myopic eyes can often be successfully treated if they are diagnosed early.

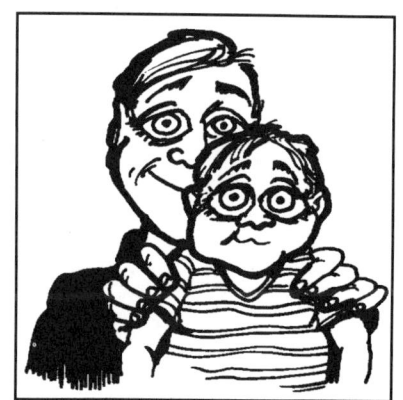

You probably don't have any diseases or problems, and the ophthalmologist makes small satisfied grunts and mmm-hmmms as he goes to the next part of his job: measuring the cornea. Besides measuring its diameter (which hasn't changed much since you were three) he measures its curvature with a keratometer, and its thickness with a device called a pachymeter. He may also run a test for dryness.

Which Eye is the Boss?

Finally, the doc will find out which of your eyes is dominant. Having read the next chapter of this book, you will probably already have determined whether you can be satisfied with RK in just one eye, and if so, which eye.

More often than not, your dominant eye is on the same side as your dominant hand. Try this test: hold out your hands with palms outward as if you were fending off a large, friendly, soaking wet dog—with thumbs and fingers overlapping so as to form a small peephole. Sight through it at a distant point, and keep watching the distant point

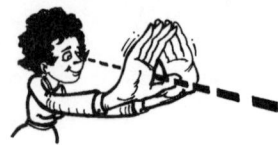

as you bring the peephole up to your face. The peephole will end up in front of your dominant eye.

Ophthalmologists can be ingenious at finding the dominant eye. Sometimes neither eye is strongly dominant, and you may have a challenge picking the leader. If it turns out you are the visual equivalent of ambidextrous, you may consider things like which eye you use to back up the car, or for a target sport.

Getting The RK Okay

While all this is going on you get to know your ophthalmologist a bit. Your ophthalmologist also gets to know you a little, as well as your eyes. Possibly he has reason to think you are not a good candidate for radial keratotomy. Some such "contra-indications":

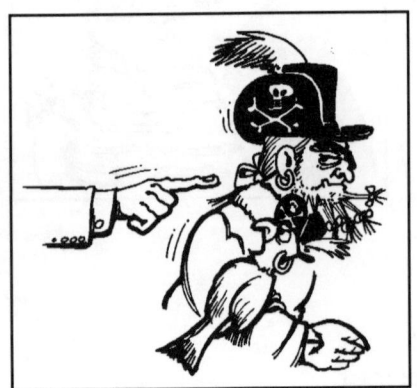

If you only have one good eye, it should never be operated on unless it is absolutely necessary, so RK is out.

If one eye is perfectly good but not being used properly—a "weak eye" that may have a tendency to turn inward or outward—that should be made right prior to RK, or any surgery that might challenge the eyes' ability to work together.

RK requires a healthy cornea. Scars or thin spots caused by injuries or diseases in the past may complicate the picture. There's an ocular form of herpes which often recurs over and over; if you've had that you probably can't have RK.

If your cornea is already very flat, and your nearsightedness results from an unusually long eye, RK may not be able to help. This rarely is a problem.

If the first trace of age-related cataract (cloudy natural lens) is evident—whoa! In cataract surgery they take your natural lens out and replace it with a plastic one, of customized power. That artificial lens will probably take care of your nearsightedness, so there's no need for RK.

And You Have to Deal with Pressure

Your intraocular pressure may be too low. If so, and you neglected to mention a marijuana habit, make sure you mention it now. And some people, commonly young women, just happen to have a low intraocular pressure.

The surgeon may have turned up some serious problem, or some minor thing like an eyelid disorder which will need to be corrected before RK.

You may be too severely nearsighted for RK to be likely to give you 20/20 or even 20/100. If under 40, you'll probably get no more than 5 or 6 diopters of correction, so if you're a -8 going in you may still be a -3 afterward, a result that you may or may not feel is worth the bother. RK can tackle higher degrees of myopia in older patients, whose corneas respond more to the operation. And some high-myopia-haters do use RK to become low myopes. We've got a whole chapter coming up on high myopia and the several methods of correcting it.

On the other hand, your nearsightedness may be so mild that the doctor will think you should save your money. You might counter by suggesting he take your low myopia into account, and offer you a lower price! (Smile when you say that.) If you have a measly diopter and a half of myopia, but would like to have hawkeye vision, your chances of getting it with RK are good.

You may have more astigmatism than the surgeon feels she is likely to be able to correct. Low astigmatism can be handled by most of the more experienced RK ophthalmologists, but high astigmatism, as we'll see, is still a real challenge for refractive surgery, with only a few surgeons specializing in this area.

Old Enough to Vote for RK?

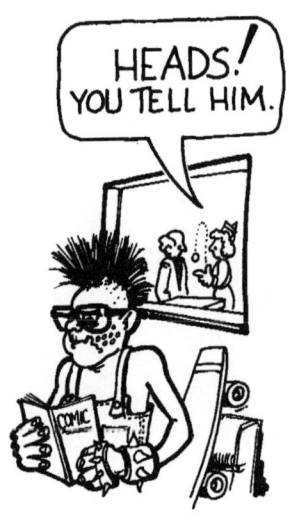

You may be too young. Eighteen is usually the minimum, and many doctors think that's pushing it. It's important that your eyes have stabilized, and are not still changing as you grow. Some eyes keep changing longer, so the doc will want two refractions done a year apart to confirm that your myopia is stable—call your optician for this paperwork. And the doc will ask whether you have thoroughly investigated contact-lenses.

You aren't too old, as long as you and your eyes are in superb health. In fact, as we've mentioned, older patients can get higher degrees of myopia corrected. However, older people are more prone to over-respond to the operation, and come away farsighted, and older folks hate farsightedness most of all, so most doctors play it safe and use a less powerful operation.

Some surgeons worry about performing RK on yoga enthusiasts, people who exercise in inversion boots, and serious weightlifters, who sometimes get increased effect or other surprising results. Very skinny young men with protruding Adam's-apples are also said to get more effect than would be expected. Young women with low intraocular pressure get very little effect. If you fall into one of these categories, discuss it with your doctor.

The Psychological Psyde

That pretty well covers the medical barriers to RK. There is also a psychological side to each human being and his vision, of course, and the doc must try to be sure that here too, all is well. Does this patient understand the decision he or she is making?

If you have told the ophthalmologist that you actually don't mind wearing glasses, and just want RK to be stylish, he'll talk you out of it. If you haven't given contact lenses a thorough trial, he may suggest that you do before resorting to surgery.

Most surgeons also discourage patients who have unrealistic expectations (who say things like "I just know I'll get 20/20 vision"), or who seem to be too immature or irrational to make a complex decision. This is a matter for mature, responsible adults who are competent enough to assume the consequences of their own decisions.

Both Feet Firmly on the Ground?

Above all: do you understand that nothing is guaranteed? Even if 95% of patients like you are satisfied, that leaves five percent who aren't. And if only one patient in ten or twenty thousand loses the use of an eye, somebody has to be that one patient. No matter how certain your doc is that it won't be you, he has to admit that it just possibly might. And so do you. We'll discuss the odds of success and the risks in chapters 11 and 12.

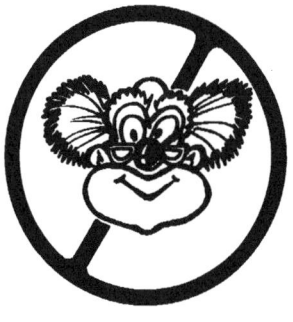

The doctor will describe RK and touch on most of the points this book covers, and quite possibly hit something we missed, so listen closely. You'll be given some leaflets on the procedure, and asked to watch a short video. Those doctors who most strongly believe in informing their patients will give you a copy of this book to read. Then you should have another chance to ask questions. Don't be shy or fearful about wasting the doctor's time, because you will be paying for all of this. The operation goes quickly; the examinations, recovery check-ups, conversations and planning are how your surgeon earns his fee.

Be sure to discuss with the doc any point we have raised that leaves you more baffled than enlightened. Put markers in the book as you go. And as a favor to your dear author, if the doc hasn't read it please ask him to. We would welcome his comments.

The ophthalmologist is risking his insurability and a little of his sanity every time he accepts a surgical patient for any procedure. He has the right to refuse to perform RK on anybody. You also have the right to choose another surgeon, with no hard feelings. Ask for the names of others to contact. Ask the doctor to describe his experience.

If you sense that the doctor is at all doubtful about you as an RK patient, find out if such is the case. Several surgeons have told me that the patients about whom they feel strange misgivings are often the patients who end up dissatisfied. Doctors are only human; like all of us they have hunches and feel "bad vibes". Give the doctor's sixth sense, and your own, a chance to be heard from.

Congratulations!

If the ophthalmologist is satisfied that you are a good candidate for RK and that you know what you are doing, he will give you an "informed consent" form to fill out. This document will list every risk and disappointment that the surgeon can think of, and require you to acknowledge them.

If you decide to proceed with RK (we'll discuss that decision in chapter 13) the next thing on the agenda is to plan your surgery. One eye or two? Four incisions or eight? If you've chosen an experienced doctor, you can trust him or her to make the many lesser decisions for you, but you certainly should know what's going to be done and why. And as we'll see, less is more!

There's a sign in a Seattle bookstore that reads, "War is Peace. Hate is Love. Ignorance is Strength." Sarcastic, but it's a good point. You now have a better understanding of your eyes than 99% of the people will ever have, so at last we can look at the remarkable choices you now have the knowledge to make, in hopes of strengthening your body in an astonishing way.

Two Eyes, Two Visions   7

Ever since I had my RK, I get a little surprise every now and then. I'll happen to rub my right eye, or cover it with my hand—and suddenly, I'm nearsighted! Since only my right eye was operated on, looking through the left eye gives me a reminder of how my vision used to be. When I reopen my right eye, everything snaps back into focus.

I am one of the thousands of mildly or moderately-nearsighted people who have had only one eye RK'd, or have had the second eye only partially corrected, yet see just as well as if both eyes were equally sharp. It won't work for everybody. In fact, probably only a minority of nearsighted people can enjoy it. But for us lucky ones it's wonderful.

It's called *monovision*. What a weird word! Sounds like what a cyclops would have. All it means is that only one eye has good distance vision, yet one sees as well as if both eyes were equal.

Knowing that you can get excellent vision with one eye left nearsighted makes RK extremely attractive. If one eye will do the trick, you're looking at half the cost, half the inconvenience —half of all the negative things, but still all of the benefit you would get if both eyes were operated. Wow!

Preserving "The Revenge of the Nearsighted"

Of course, the main reason to leave one eye nearsighted is to save that one advantage of myopia: the protection it gives you against presbyopia, the loss of near vision that the 20/20 eye experiences in middle age. The surplus power of the myopic eye makes the lens' accommodative power unnecessary, so the nearsighted person will always be able to read just by removing his or her glasses.

You may have had a great-uncle who never needed glasses, in youth or in age, for reading or for distance. This lucky gent probably had two mismatched eyes, one 20/20 and the other nearsighted. It happens, rarely. It's going to get a lot more common.

The Contact Connection

In recent years many contact-lens wearers have been reaching the presbyopic age of 45 or thereabouts, and finding that they cannot read with their contacts in place. It's more of a nuisance for them than for spectacle-wearing nearsighted folks, who merely take off their glasses—it's not so easy to take off contacts whenever you need to read something. Some such people get reading glasses to wear over their contacts, and a few find professionals who are skilled at the specialized art of fitting bifocal contact lenses. But increasingly, people are just using a contact in one eye, for distance, and leaving the other eye nearsighted for reading.

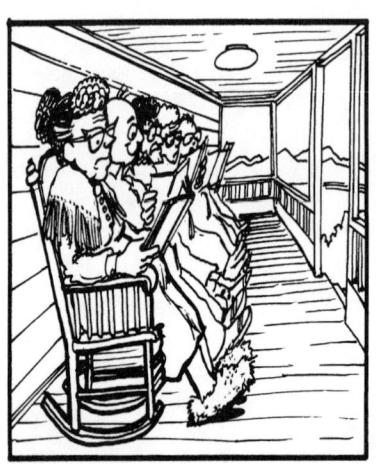

Nearsighted people can usually read without glasses in senior years. Find the myope in this picture

"We call it 'contact-lens monovision'", optometrist Dr. Bob Miller told me. "It just growed, like Topsy. There's no literature on it, and the industry doesn't promote it—patients just discover that it works. I always suggest that people try it before looking at bifocal contact lenses."

A Lovely Couple: RK and Monovision Look So Good Together

One of the most scientific of the early RK surgeons, Dr. Michael Deitz of Kansas City, Kansas, was among the first to emphasize that many RK patients are happy with only one eye corrected, if they are patient enough to give it a chance. Unfortunately, it takes some people several months to adjust to it.

Many people assume that having two differently-focused eyes would be unbearable. For some people, it is, but many people have no problem with a difference of two to three diopters—which means that one eye can be left nearsighted enough to save you from the need for reading glasses in the presbyopic years.

Times Of Our Lives, Eyewise

Visual Life-Cycles:

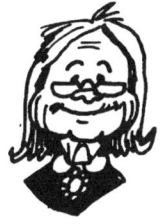

20/20 seer needs reading glasses in middle-age and senior years

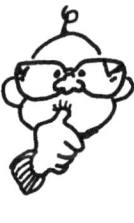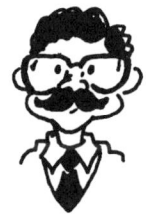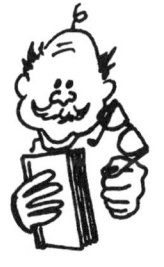

Over-2 D-nearsighted fella can still read in senior years by taking off glasses

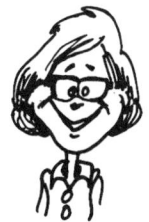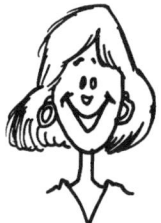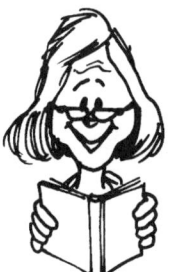

This myopic lady has both eyes RK'd successfully, so like the 20/20 people she needs reading glasses later

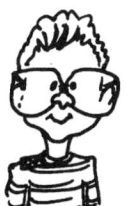

Monovision! This guy was nearsighted, had one eye RK'd. Other eye still myopic for easy near vision.

A Lifelong Bare-eyed Looker!

Living with monovision isn't a matter of being able to tolerate a half-blurry view. The toleration involved is subconscious: the brain shuts out the blurry image and "sees" only the sharp one in detail. The brain's ability to do such things is impressive, and is well known to ophthalmologists.

Monovision Works!

Your author's brain, a somewhat underpowered '53 model (slightly the worse for wear—some crazy teenager owned it back in the late sixties) is very tolerant of monovision. It ignores the blurry image that my moderately-nearsighted left eye sends it when I'm looking far, and the even blurrier image produced by my right eye when I'm reading. For a brain that can't work a Rubik's cube or avoid burning a TV dinner two tries out of three, this seems like quite a feat!

The matter of depth perception is hard to pin down. The part of depth perception that is supplied by using two eyes, called stereo-acuity, may be decreased, although it may be that the image from a mildly myopic eye is still good enough for this purpose. Some people with one corrected eye say that their depth perception is slightly diminished, and will wear a contact lens for demanding activities such as baseball or hunting.

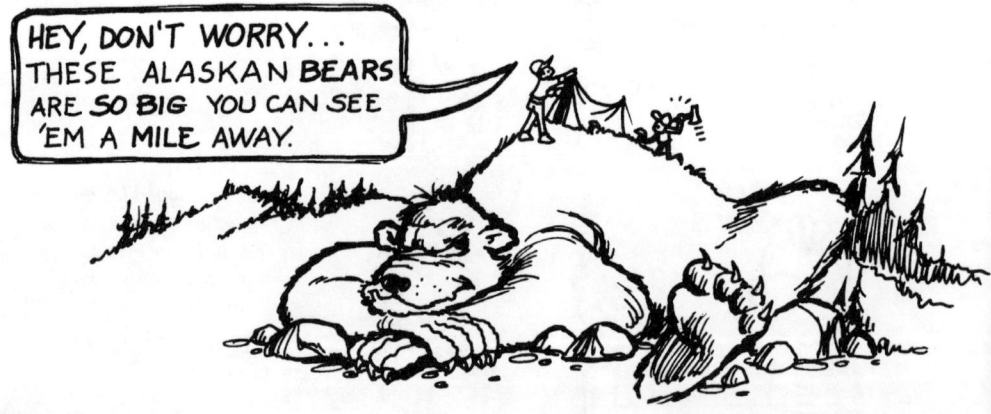

When I look far the blurry image is perfectly fused with the sharp one, and I don't see the blurry one at all except sometimes late at night, when I'm really bushed. If I hold the book close when I read, the blurry image from my RK'd eye does not fuse; it remains separate. I see the page double and simply ignore one of the images, not even aware that it's there. If I hold the book a bit farther out, the two images fuse together and the blurry one disappears.

But Not for Wayne Gretsky

The only sport in which my nearsighted left eye is a nuisance is hockey: when skating backward, you have to look over your shoulder with one eye, to see where you are going. When I look over my left shoulder with my left eye, I'm still nearsighted! Since most of the guys I collide with are bigger than I am and seem to be equipped with extra sets of elbows, this can hurt.

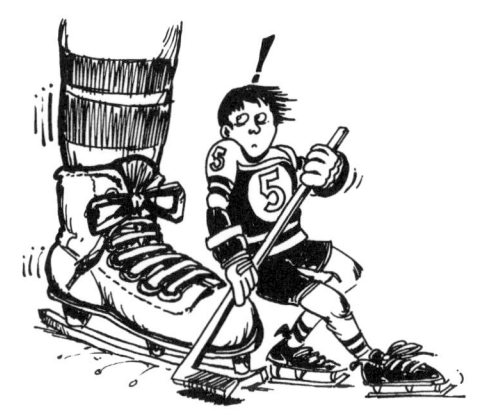

A Lifelong Bare-eyed Looker?

If you are mildly nearsighted, there's a good chance that you will be happy with only one eye RK'd. You may be able to prove this to yourself in advance by wearing a lens over your dominant eye only—although a contact lens should be used rather than glasses. Glasses shrink the image size, and the difference in size annoys the brain much more than any difference in focus.

If you have a pair of contact lenses, try wearing just one of them, in your dominant eye. You may find yourself adjusting to this very readily. If so— if you find that your dominant eye automatically takes over for distance, and your uncorrected eye takes over for near—congratulations! In a sense, you are already halfway finished with the RK program: one eye is all set, one to go. Plus, with one myopic "extra-strength" eye for permanent near vision, you're a potential life-long bare-eyed looker!

However, most people need time to adjust to monovision, and you may not be willing to wear a contact lens in one eye for very long. So many patients will not discover monovision until after their first eye is operated. Dr. Deitz finds that patients who, one month after their first RK, are determined that the other eye must also be done, often are less positive after three months, and are quite willing to "listen to reason" after six months. If they wait a full year, they usually lose all interest in having their second eye operated.

A Real Eye-Opener

It's a good idea to have a cycloplegic examination after the first RK. The accommodation-paralyzing cycloplegic drops show the younger patient what life will be like at fifty-five, and how nice it is to have some myopia in one eye. The discovery that with the RK'd eye it will be impossible to read without glasses is quite startling—no matter how often you are told this, seeing it for yourself has far more impact.

Of course, some people simply can't tolerate even a two-diopter difference between their eyes. If you remain unhappy with the unilateral RK, perhaps you are one of the ones who just can't be happy with monovision.

The RK-and-a-Half Approach

If you are moderately nearsighted—say, four diopters—you will probably need the second eye at least partly corrected. After the first eye has been done, give monovision a chance. Perhaps you will be happy most of the time, and only need a contact lens in the unoperated eye for demanding activities. But if you really don't like having one eye left with those four diopters of myopia, don't assume you need a full correction in that second eye. Maybe a partial correction will satisfy you—perhaps leaving two diopters of myopia in the second eye, enough for lifelong reading. You can do some testing to find out.

Wear a contact lens with enough power to simulate a half-strength RK (leaving about -2 D) in your unoperated eye until you are sure that you can tolerate a partial correction. Don't try it when you have a cold or flu, or when you're exhausted—the brain has times when it's in no mood to tolerate anything new.

"Why Don't You Wear Glasses Like My Other Grampa, Grampa?"

If you are comfortable with a half-strength RK in your second (probably your non-dominant) eye, that's great! That will leave enough myopia in one eye to prevent near-vision loss in the presbyopic years.

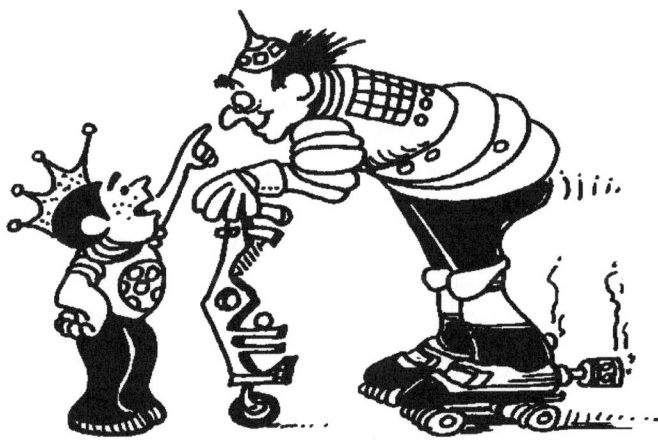

In fact, about -2 D or -2.50 D myopia in one eye is ideal—that's just enough for lifelong easy reading. We have seen that the more nearsighted you are, the closer you must hold a book to see it. With five diopters of myopia you can focus well only out to eight inches, whereas with two and a half diopters you can focus out to sixteen inches. Plus, the less nearsighted your nearsighted eye is, the better vision your senior self will have in the whole middle range, from sixteen inches to twenty feet. So for the -4 D or -5 D myope, there is an advantage to having the second eye half-corrected rather than left as-is. Certainly, it's worth taking considerable trouble to find out if you can handle a partial correction in the second eye.

This all seems like an awful pain, but the reward is worth it! The average American lives thirty years with presbyopia. Unless you have at least one eye that's two or three diopters myopic, you will have to put on a pair of glasses every time you need to read small print—not just a book in your easy chair at home, but also a price tag, a menu, a telephone book, a road map. This is hard for a nearsighted person to imagine; it's a good idea to ask your ophthalmologist to simulate it for you with lenses, or with cycloplegia after your first RK. It's no fun.

Respect Older People, Like the One You'll Become

It almost seems that we humans hate our own future selves, to judge by all the things we do that they will have to pay for. You might choose good distance vision over good near vision if you had to choose one or the other, but the opportunity to have both offers an unusual chance to do something nice for yourself! Take the trouble to preserve some nearsightedness in one eye so that in the future you will not have to put on glasses to see close up.

Many surgeons prefer to operate on the non-dominant eye first; the theory is that it's more forgivable to accidentally undercorrect or overcorrect that eye, and the results of that first operation will give clues to how much your corneas respond, aiding the doc in his encore operation on your more important eye. This consideration is probably less crucial than the value of keeping your non-dominant eye for reading in those later decades. Unless you are positive that you cannot tolerate monovision, you should consider having your dominant eye corrected first. Although for some people it doesn't matter, for most the dominant eye is best for distant vision and should be given the full correction.

It may be that you can't handle any significant difference between your eyes. At least you'll know you tried. Too many RK patients never give it a thought.

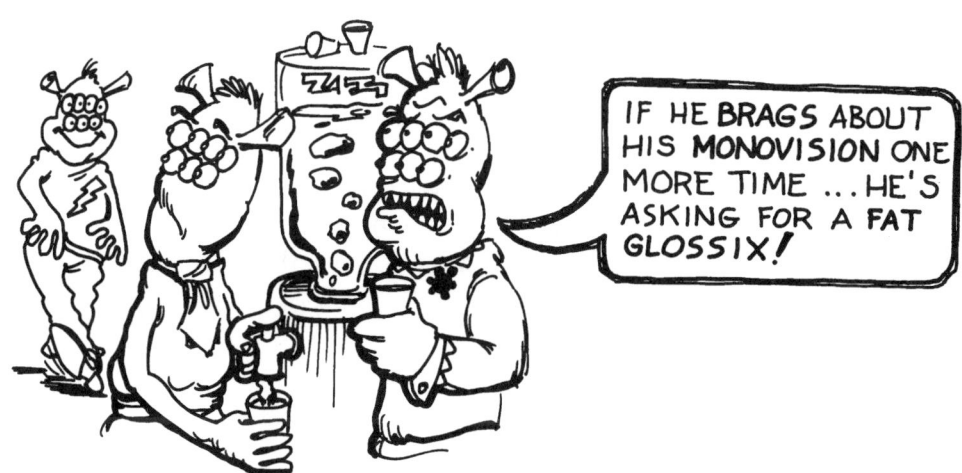

The Great Monovisionaries

Some ophthalmologists are big believers in monovision RK, and try to persuade their often-recalcitrant patients to give it a chance. My own surgeon, Dr. Grendahl, is such a one, for which I'm eternally grateful. But some don't promote it at all—because it's a fairly new discovery, better known to optometrists than to ophthalmologists, because it is contrary to the dogma that mismatched eyes are uncomfortable (which is true of higher degrees of mismatch), and often because they've had too many patients who refused to consider the advantages of it.

Whether your doctor favors monovision or not, you should pursue it. Especially if you're a low myope of 2 or 3 diopters, make sure you can't enjoy single-eye correction before you go for that second-eye operation. Even the day before the second eye is scheduled: if you're suddenly not positive that you need it, hold off!

Less is More

I guess I've made this point as forcefully as I can without making a nuisance of myself. But stressing the one-of-each advantage is part of the smart approach to RK: a cautious, minimalist approach, designed to get the benefits of this amazing operation while taking as few risks as possible.

Next: the Plan.

The RK Candidate Plans the Campaign

8

"Well, you have no problems that would rule out RK," says your ophthalmologist.

"So I'm a good candidate?" you ask.

The ophthalmologist's answer is going to depend mainly on how nearsighted you are and how much astigmatism you have. If you're only mildly myopic, say 2 diopters, and have no astigmatism, he or she may say something like:

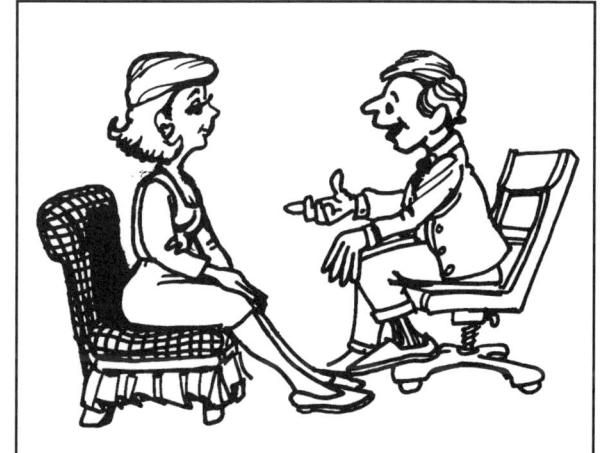

"Yes, you would have about a 90% to 95% chance of coming away with 20/40 vision, good enough to drive without glasses. And about a 75% chance of 20/20 or better. Also, you may be happy with only one eye operated—let's test you for monovision tolerance."

If, on the other hand, you're a young man or woman with seven or eight diopters of myopia, he might say: "No, you're not an ideal candidate. RK could only offer you about a 55% chance of reaching 20/40 and a 30% chance of 20/20. If you were twenty years older you'd have better odds of getting enough correction, but as it is you should expect to still need glasses after the operation, although not thick ones like you wear now."

This is a good time to find out just why the RK prospects are better for the low and moderate myopes than for the highly nearsighted folks.

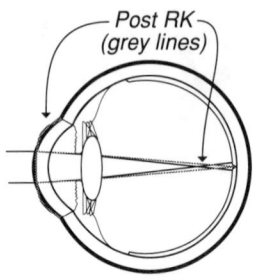

*Mild Myopia
Only slight flattening of
Cornea required.*

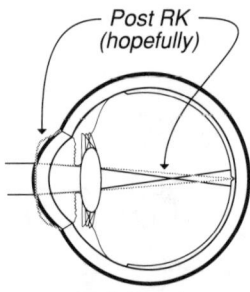

*High Myopia
Major flattening
of Cornea required
(exaggerated view)*

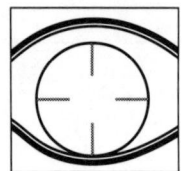

*Low Myopia:
4 or 8 incisions*

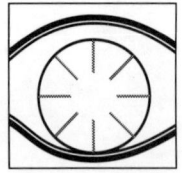

*Moderate and High
Myopia: 8 incisions*

Nobody Said It Would be Fair

The more myopic you are, the farther in front of your retina the image is being focused, so the more your cornea needs to be flattened in order to relax its focusing and put that image back where it belongs. And more cornea-flattening requires more cornea-incising.

Other than waiting until the patient is older, there are only three ways of making the operation more effective, to cause more flattening: use more incisions, deeper incisions, or longer incisions which crowd in closer in the center, leaving a smaller clear central zone.

Eight Is Enough

The most obvious way of increasing the flattening is to add more incisions: instead of four the doc can use eight, and get about 30% more effect. He can use sixteen, but that will add only another 10% of effect—not much, considering that the "insult" to the cornea is doubled, with twice the soreness and other post-op annoyances. Also, there is more likelihood of starburst and glare, with all those microscopic scars to diffuse light.

Several years ago, sixteen and even thirty-two incisions were frequently used for highly myopic cases. Nowadays, patients who need such heroic measures are usually discouraged from trying RK. Many patients did get satisfactory results, but too many wound up with complications, and wished they'd never ventured. In addition to the other problems inherent in doing so much cutting, most surgeons find that after the first eight cuts, the cornea becomes so flexible that it's hard to get the depth right on any further incisions.

Some surgeons do use twelve incisions or even sixteen, and strongly believe they can do so safely, but the majority draw the line at eight.

Cutting Deep

Deeper incisions also increase the flattening. Instead of cutting 85% of the way through the cornea, surgeons can go as deep as 95%. The main reason they don't is fear of perforating the cornea.

When this happens, the knife cuts through the fragile endothelium (the cornea's inner lining) and a tiny bead of eye fluid appears. The almost-microscopic puncture heals quickly and usually causes no problems, but this does increase the remote risk of infection inside the eye. Also, too-deep cuts may cause the operation's result to be unstable, a problem we'll examine later.

And when the surgeon cuts this deep, the effect becomes more unpredictable. So most doctors try to keep their cuts in the 85%-through range.

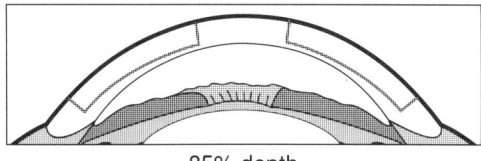
85% depth

Cross-section of cornea with 85%-depth incisions

Cutting it Close to the Central Zone

The third and most important method of increasing the effect of RK is to extend the incisions in closer to the center of the cornea, toward the central optical zone, the crucial middle part you actually look through when you look at something. Refractive surgeons call it the "clear zone" because the incisions never cross it—they radiate away from it across the outer cornea, through which only peripheral vision is seen.

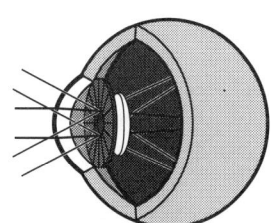

Incisions go in the outer parts of the cornea—peripherial-vision country.

Flattening the central cornea is the point of the whole exercise, however, and the closer in toward the center the incisions go, the more it flattens. Dramatically so: bringing the incisions in a measly half-millimeter closer may add a whole diopter of correction.

This is the most useful method of adjusting the intended effect of RK. Many surgeons never vary the depth of their incisions, and rarely use more than eight cuts. Other than using four or six incisions instead of eight, their method of controlling the degree of effect is varying the size of the uncut central zone, using a tiny 3-mllimeter zone when maximum effect is required, and up to 5mm for the mildest myopia.

So for most surgeons, the most powerful RK consists of eight cuts at 85-90% depth, with a 3mm central clear optical zone. This will correct about five or six diopters of myopia, depending on the patient's age. (Dr. James Salz cites this rule of thumb: RK can usually correct about 2.5 diopters plus a tenth of the patient's age in diopters. For a thirty-year-old patient, that would be 5.5 diopters of correction; at age fifty, 7.5 diopters.)

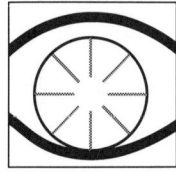

3mm optical zone

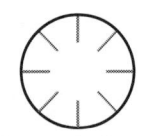

5mm optical zone

If life were fair, RK would be just as likely to succeed for the high myope as for the mildly nearsighted person. Do you suppose that somewhere at the center of the galaxy, there is a planet where life is fair? Me neither.

Ancient Chinese Curse: May You Live in Interesting Times

The highly nearsighted person (over six diopters) has an "interesting time" with RK: more chance of undercorrection, of still having to wear glasses—albeit much thinner ones, and probably not all the time. Also, the more powerful the surgery the greater the chances of experiencing the occasional side-effects we'll be discussing later.

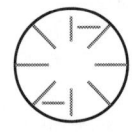

Mild Astigmatism RK

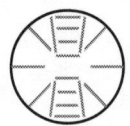

Severe Astigmatism RK

The chances of success are also diminished if the nearsightedness is combined with high astigmatism. While mild astigmatism can usually be cured by adding a few small incisions to the RK operation, astigmatism over three or four diopters is likely to decrease the chances of success considerably, as we'll see in our astigmatism chapter.

Even without the added problem of astigmatism, high myopes have much less chance of freedom from glasses after RK. On the other hand, it's true that the more highly nearsighted patients, even if not perfectly corrected, stand to gain the most dramatic improvement in visual realism, to a full-sized image free of the "barrel-distortion" they endure with glasses. They are almost sure of being able to read comfortably, or use a computer, without glasses. The fact that they will probably not get a full correction does have the advantage of preserving near-vision through middle and senior years. In fact, every surgeon who has read this chapter has pointed out that some of his or her most ecstatic patients were high myopes who did not achieve 20/40 vision. We'll scratch our heads over that in our high-myopia chapter.

How Many Sticks of Dynamite, Sundance?

So the surgeon adjusts the power of his operation by adjusting the number of cuts, and how close they come in toward the center—that is, the diameter of the central clear zone. Several formulas have been devised to determine the best specifications for each degree of nearsightedness, and these formulas have been worked into tables and personal-computer programs. These "nomograms", as they are called, attempt to factor in every important particular about your eyes, and predict the operation most likely to achieve a given degree of cornea-flattening.

The most important factors include your degree of nearsightedness, your age, and your sex—we've mentioned that as you age you become a better RK prospect, since the older cornea seems to "stay put" better as it heals, and doesn't tend to regress as much. Among young patients, men get more effect from the same operation than women

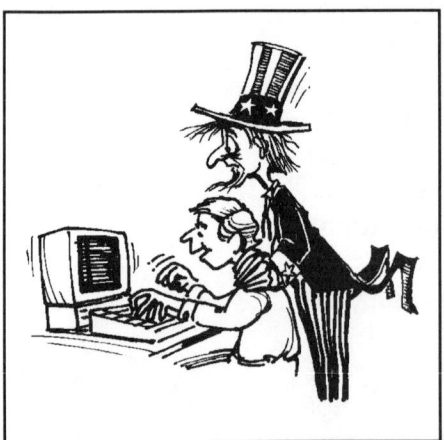

"Let's see, you're around 215 years old..."

do, but as age increases women "catch up" in this regard, and women over 40 get as much effect as men do.

The size and curvature of your cornea are factored in—larger and thicker corneas get more flattening effect—and your intraocular pressure (more pressurized eyes also respond more to the operation). With this data, the chart or computer program is able to help the surgeon decide on the particulars: the number, depth and length of the micro-incisions. (Note: it doesn't matter whether a computer or a printed table is used; the formula is what matters.)

The surgeon wants to get you as close as possible to emmetropia, the perfect focus of the 20/20 eye. He doesn't want to "undercorrect", and leave you still nearsighted, but what he wants even less is to "overcorrect", and make you farsighted.

Eventually, we hope, somebody will devise a test that will tell the doctor in advance just how much your cornea will respond to the incisions, and warn him if yours is one of the few percent that tend to overrespond. Today, no such test exists.

For Now, Use the Anti-Overcorrection Approach

In recent years, many surgeons have been taking a more cautious approach to RK. Instead of using the operation most likely to result in 20/20 vision, and accepting the fact that some patients would under-respond and remain nearsighted while others would over-respond and become farsighted, they play it on the safe side. They use a slightly less effective form of the operation—sometimes four incisions instead of eight, or a larger optical zone—and thereby tilt the odds in favor of undercorrection, and make it less likely that the patient will come away farsighted.

Of course, this means that you are more likely to be left still slightly nearsighted—at least in the first eye that is operated. These surgeons accept that likelihood, and are willing to re-operate on patients who are still nearsighted after the first operation, in hopes of getting more correction.

Dr. James Salz of Los Angeles' Cedars-Sinai Medical Center explains, "The idea of 4-incision radial keratotomy is this: It is far better to undercorrect than to overcorrect a patient, because undercorrection can usually be remedied by adding four more incisions, whereas overcorrection is very hard to fix. Once we see the response to four incisions in the first eye, we can use that result in planning the surgery in the second eye, and often get the second eye just right. Then we can go back and add four more in the first eye, if necessary. It's more trouble, but it's worth it to minimize the chances of overcorrection. After all, we're talking about the vision you'll probably have for life."

Overcorrection Can be Fun When You're Young, But...

The accommodation ability of the lens usually hides the effect of a mild overcorrection, until age 40 or so. So the surgeons find that their younger overcorrected patients are often delighted for years, even decades. Monovision patients are more tolerant of overcorrection—since only one eye is RK'd, the other will always be nearsighted for easy reading. And a slightly overcorrected eye may have sharp distance vision as long as it has accommodation. Nevertheless, it's best to take a cautious, anti-overcorrection approach.

The Lesser of Two Eyevils

Some surgeons use slightly different strategies with the same basic idea. Some, for example, prefer the original eight-incision plan, but still can do "touch-up" re-operations.

Discuss the steer-toward-undercorrection approach with your ophthalmologist. Ask whether the surgeon will be willing to do a "touch-up" operation if you are undercorrected after the first try, and what the charge for that would be. Even the most cautious surgeons do get some overcorrections, perhaps 5% to 10% of the time, but you and your doctor should try to minimize the chance of this even if it takes some extra trouble. Also, remember that not all undercorrections can be improved by re-operation, and after one re-operation attempt you have to call it quits and be content, even though you may still be undercorrected.

If you are not a simple, straightforward case—if you're over six diopters nearsighted, or have more than two or three diopters of astigmatism—and decide to go ahead anyway, make sure you and your surgeon discuss his experience in dealing with cases like yours.

Suitable for Framing: Your RK Plan

In any event, prior to the day of the operation your ophthalmologist should have a complete surgical plan that he can show you. It will begin with your prescription, and other data about your eye. Here's a totally hypothetical one:

DATA FOR RK PREDICTION
FOR RIGHT EYE:
REFRACTION: -2.25 D -.50 x 180 [You've got 2.25 diopters of nearsight, plus a negligible half-diopter of astigmatism]

SPHERICAL EQUIVALENT: -2.50 D [Your refraction, with the astigmatism averaged out and added in]

AVERAGE KERATOMETRY: 43.9 D [Your cornea's total power]

INTRAOCULAR PRESSURE: 13 [Nice and firm, like the tires on a 10-speed]

Planning

DESIRED FINAL RESULT: -.50 D [You're trying to minimize the likelihood of overcorrection by accepting a little residual myopia.]

DESIRED CHANGE IN SPHERICAL EQUIVALENT: 2.00 [The eye has 2.5 diopters of nearsightedness, but you want a half-diopter safety margin, leaving 2 diopters to be corrected.]

The plan for your operation will follow. If it's a computer printout, there may be a table showing a series of different possible plans, and the predicted correction for each. Your ophthalmologist will pick the one that feels right to him, and explain it to you. In this hypothetical case it might be either a 4-incision or an eight-incision plan—the four-cut is great because it's easier to fine-tune later if undercorected, but the eight-cut plan is preferred by many surgeons because it's more forgiving of minute variations between the incisions. Here is a hypothetical 4-incision plan:

NUMBER OF INCISIONS: 4
OPTICAL ZONE: 3.5 mm
INCISION DEPTH: 90%
PREDICTED CHANGE IN SPERICAL EQUIVALENT: 2.05 [which is almost exactly the amount of correction desired.]

If the result of your operation is precisely as predicted, you'll come out with a negligible half-diopter of myopia. The danger of overcorrection, though still present, is minimized: if your cornea over-responds by a diopter, you'll still only be half a diopter farsighted. If you underrespond, the doc may be able to fine-tune you with a touch-up operation. There is no provision for astigmatism, because in this case it's too slight to be a problem.

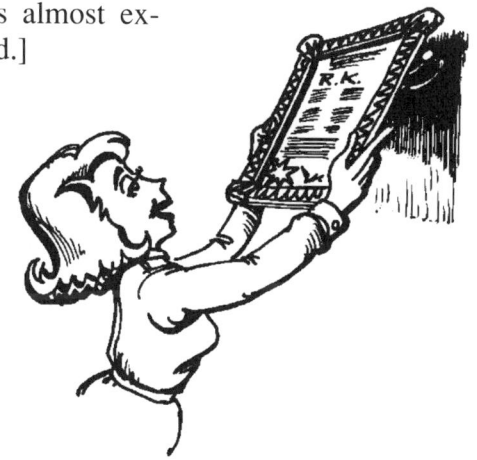

The outcome of this first operation will be used to help plan the surgery in the second eye, if both eyes are being done. For example, if the first eye is surprisingly undercorrected, a more powerful plan can be used in the second eye. Obviously, if both eyes are done the same day this opportunity to observe and modify is lost, so there should always be a waiting period between the two eyes.

The Better Part of Valor

As you can see we're taking a conservative approach to RK: One eye at a time, if possible trying to conserve some nearsightedness in one eye for near-vision in middle age, attempting to decrease the odds of overcorrection even if it means increasing the chances of undercorrection. We're not trying to be heroes, right?

Next: the RK operation.

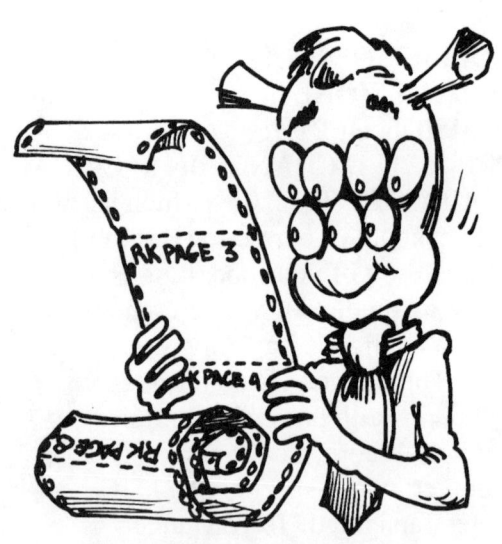

The RK Operation

9

"Did you say you'll be out this morning, John?" asked my foreman, Terry.

"Yes, I'll be getting operated on," I said.

"No kidding? Getting something removed?"

"Yeah, I hope so—nearsightedness. With luck I won't have to wear glasses after today."

I drove myself to Dr. Grendahl's building, confident that I'd be able to drive back to the shop afterward and finish up some work before taking off early in the afternoon. After all, only one eye was being operated on.

Naturally I was excited about the possibility of not having to wear glasses. Although I knew there were no guarantees, the odds looked very good. Still, I was a little apprehensive. I'd been through surgery before, but not eye surgery. The idea of watching the knife descend gave me the willies.

The doctor's assistant gave me a scrub suit and a sedative pill which I put on and in, respectively, before relaxing on a couch for a few minutes. Soon I was ushered into the outpatient surgery room, which looked like my dentist's office except (mercifully) no cute pictures of fluffy cats tacked to the ceiling. I got on the table and made bad jokes as Dr. Grendahl, a reassuringly professional surgeon, prepared to perform the radial keratotomy.

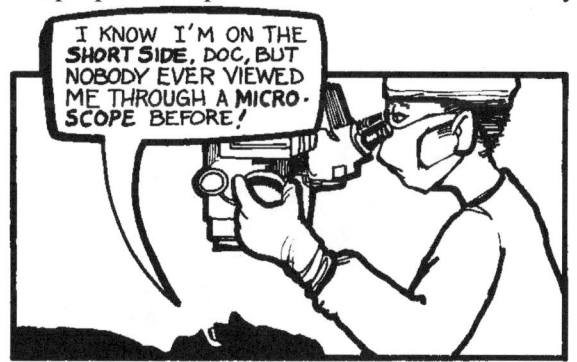

I told you they were bad

Our Hero Gets an Upgrade

Dr. Grendahl put a few drops in my eye and asked me to focus for a moment on the filament in a large light overhead, and to hold my eye steady. I noticed that my eyelid was propped open, but Diane moistened my eye for me so I didn't mind. As it turned out I couldn't see the incisions being made, which was fine with me, and thanks to the anesthetic drops I couldn't feel them either.

In a few minutes it was over. It was almost anticlimactic. "You call that an operation?" I wanted to say. Just a month before I'd had a tooth pulled, a procedure that involved three injections, wads of bloody cotton and a muscular dentist heaving on a pair of pliers. I had felt like I got my money's worth then.

As I rested in the outer room, Dr. Grendahl stopped by to ask how I felt. "Great!" I replied. "Not a bit sore. I guess I'll drive on back to the office."

"Wait until the anesthetic wears off, and see how you feel," he advised with a knowing smile. "Keep that patch on tonight—I'll take it off when you come in tomorrow morning. Here's a prescription for some painkillers."

A few minutes later the anesthetic wore off. Feeling like the loser after the referee stops the fight, I called a cab for a ride home.

> *Remember:*
> *No surgeon can guarantee his or her results. No patient can be certain of a good result. Be sure to read the next three chapters!*

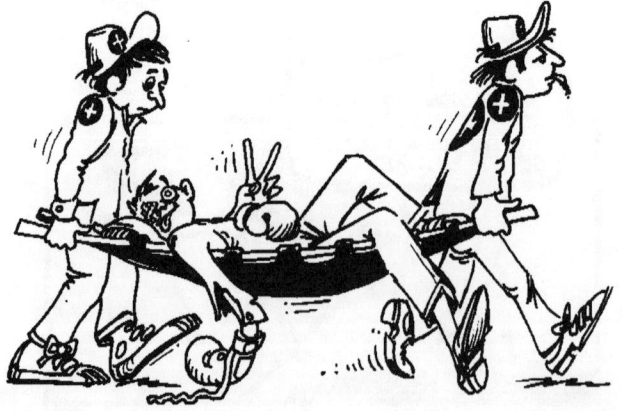

On the Day of Your Radial K

The following description of the RK operation is by no means a surgical guide or a precise technique, just a general outline so you'll know what to expect. To the surgeons it seems too short. They know and debate dozens of fine points of technique, equipment, and pharmacology. They finesse and "put a little English on it" at every stage. Compared to the mental and manual gymnastics that the surgeon goes through, this description is pretty simplified.

On the day of the operation you'll probably arrive at the ophthalmologist's office or surgicenter feeling excited, apprehensive and a little hungry, having skipped a meal. You haven't worn contact lenses for several weeks, or used any drugs without clearing them with your surgeon. You may undergo a walletectomy at this point; for many patients handing the check to the receptionist is the most painful part of the whole procedure. Then you'll probably be given a sedative (not because of the forementioned shock), and may be asked to don a scrub suit like surgeons wear.

Just when you are ready to fall asleep in your waiting room chair, the doctor's assistant will bring you into the operating room, where you can flop on the table and get comfortable while the doc fidgets with his operating microscope—a double-barreled magnification device through which your eye appears to be the size of an orange. He'll position the microscope precisely above the eye and spend some time getting your head comfortably positioned with the plane of your iris exactly horizontal. Except for that eye, the rest of you will be draped off with a lightweight sheet.

> ### *Before RK:*
> *Don't:*
> *Use marijuana*
> *Wear contact lenses*
> *Drink alcohol*
> *Use eye cosmetics*
>
> *Do:*
> *Use eyedrops provided by doctor*
> *Wash face thoroughly*
> *Check these instructions and all other important points with your surgeon.*

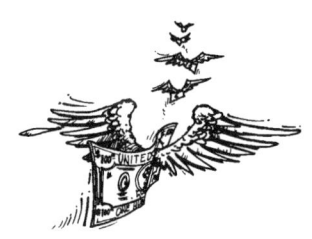

Gain but No Pain

Now it's time for anesthesia. Most ophthalmologists use nothing more than a few drops of topical anesthetic on the surface of the eye, which numbs it completely. More drops are added during the course of the operation; they keep your eye moist and unfeeling until it's all over.

Some surgeons do inject a local anesthetic, similar to novocaine—this has the advantage of immobilizing the eye by paralyzing the little muscles that move it, and it also prevents you from feeling any pinching or pressure from the forceps that will be used to hold your eye steady. But the added hazards of this type of anesthesia are considerable, so it is rarely used for RK.

For extremely nervous patients general anesthesia can be used, in a hospital operating room, but that's pretty rare—for one thing, it's too expensive. Also, the patient's active participation is lost if he's in cloudland. Once patients understand the untraumatic nature of the surgery, they realize they don't need to be knocked cold for it.

Many surgeons provide nitrous oxide if the patient desires it. This "laughing gas" is not really necessary, but it does make the whole thing more enjoyable.

A Few More Preliminaries

Next, the surgeon needs to mark the visual axis—the central point of the cornea. This is the hub of your visual universe, and the ophthalmologist wants it to be the center of the central optical zone where no incisions may intrude. He'll need your help to find it.

You may be asked to look at the coiled filament in the operating microscope light, or sometimes a tiny red bulb. As you stare at it, the surgeon can see its reflection on your cornea. He uses that

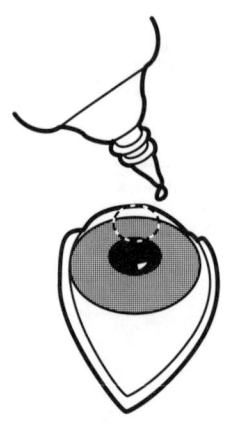

My favorite anesthetic: you don't count backwards and you don't roll over.

The RK Operation

reflection to determine the precise location of the visual axis, which he proceeds to mark with a gentle, temporary indentation. Your assistance in holding your eye very still is needed here, so think peaceful thoughts for the next few minutes.

Now the surgeon uses a little round marker to delineate the central zone into which no incisions are allowed. If he is using a 3.5mm optical clear zone, he'll use a marker just that size—that's about an eighth of an inch in diameter. He centers this little ring on the visual-axis mark he just made, and presses it gently. He will probably use another marker with little radiating spokes to mark where the incisions will go, and possibly yet another marker to help locate the position of additional transverse incisions to correct astigmatism, if necessary. All of these markers leave impressions that remain visible until the surgery is complete, and then fade away.

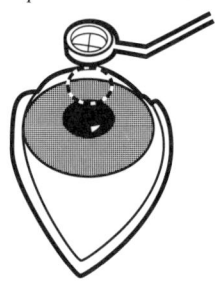

Optical-zone marker

Incision Precision

Now the surgeon may double-check the measurements he made earlier of your cornea's thickness, by touching it with a little probe wired to a meter which uses waves of ultrasound—almost like a depthfinder on a sportfishing boat. The cornea's thickness must be measured at many different locations, until the surgeon is positive of its thickness to within ten microns—that's ten millionths of a meter. Since your cornea is around 600 microns thick, that's fairly precise.

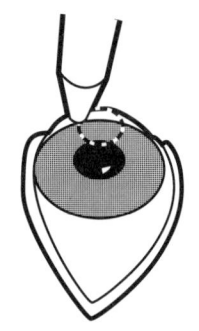

Testing Cornea thickness

Knowing exactly how thick your cornea is, the surgeon can now set the blade on his knife. However far the tiny sliver of diamond protrudes past the twin "footplates", that's how deep each incision will be. The surgeon needs to have absolute faith in both his depth measurements and his blade setting, so he may spend more time at this than he spends on the actual operation. Although these knives cost two or three thousand dollars apiece, they are not always perfectly calibrated, and the surgeon will always double-check the setting under his microscope.

Half a Millimeter Deep: That's Microsurgery!

Now all is ready for the incisions. The nurse applies another drop of anesthetic, and the doctor dabs the cornea lightly to dry it off and make the incision marks clearly visible. Gently holding the eye steady with a small instrument in his left hand, he carefully inserts the blade into the cornea until the footplates rest against the surface, and then makes the incision. Some surgeons start the cuts at the outer edge of the cornea and cut inward to the optical zone, but most start at the optical zone mark and cut out toward the edge of the cornea.

A four-incision RK being completed. The incisions are almost invisible 12 hours later; after 3 years it's hard to find 'em with a microscope.

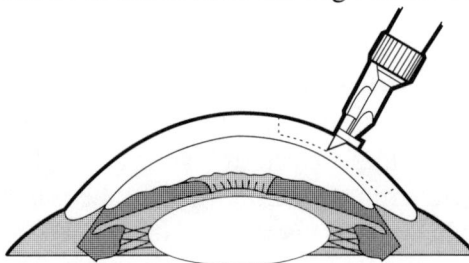

Cross-section showing depth of RK incision

The surgeon is holding the eye steady, so you can just relax. If you move your eye suddenly, it may jerk a bit and cause an imperfect incision. The trouble this will cause will probably not be serious, but try to avoid it. Don't worry if you can't resist the urge to blink; but remember the assistant is keeping the eye moist for you, and that the whole thing will be over in a few more minutes.

Depending on the amount of effect that is desired, the number of incisions can be four, six, or eight. Some doctors still occasionally use sixteen incisions (in high-myopia cases), but they do the surgery in two stages with a month or more of healing time in between.

Since the cornea is considerably thicker toward the outer rim, the outer part of each incision can be made deeper. This "peripheral redeepening" is sometimes done to increase the operation's effect in high-myopia cases.

Is It Over Already?

In less time than it takes to tell, the remaining incisions are completed and their depth is checked. You might think it would be harrowing to watch the knife at work in your very own personal eye, but because the incisions are not over the pupil, you can't actually watch the action. In fact, between the doctor's reassuring manner, the topical anesthetic and the sedative, RK may be less nerve-wracking than having your teeth cleaned.

If there is mild astigmatism to be corrected as well as nearsightedness, additional incisions are done. These are usually short (2 or 3mm) transverse incisions placed in the steep meridian, the axis of the cornea where it is more strongly curved than elsewhere. These tiny cuts cause the steep parts of the cornea to flatten some more, and hopefully correct the astigmatism.

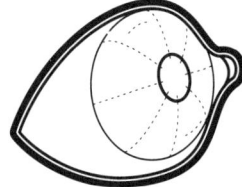

Horizontal lines are for astigmatism.
Note: *These incisions are almost invisible, and soon disappear.*

When all the incisions are completed, they may be cleaned—"irrigated"—if necessary to remove microscopic debris. Possibly the real reason for this is to trickle some water into your ear, which helps you wake up—some of us get pretty groggy from the tranquilizers. A few drops of antibiotic are then applied; you'll be given a supply of these drops to use in the coming weeks.

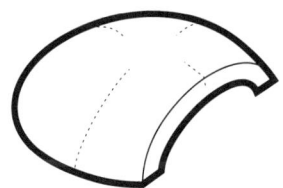

Cutaway view of cornea after eight-incision RK. The incisions are about 85 to 90 percent through the cornea.

You may notice that your vision is already much sharper. Just as you are getting interested in this, the doc will probably slap a patch over your eye (although some don't feel a patch is necessary). Then he'll shoo you out to the waiting room where you can rest while the anesthetic wears off and your eye starts to feel like it's full of sand.

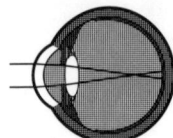 *Before RK*
 The RK Effect on the cornea, exaggerated
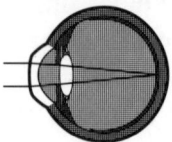 *Post-RK, hopefully*

Are We Having Fun Yet?

So that's what the RK operation is like. It may take less time to undergo RK than it takes to read about it—fifteen or twenty minutes, of which only a few minutes are spent making the incisions. And you don't have to be especially heroic to endure it, since RK is almost painless, with only mild discomfort from the eyelid being held open and sometimes a slight tugging sensation. It helps if you have the ability to be calm and helpful in unusual circumstances, because the patient's help is needed in keeping the eye still. Hopefully, having read this book you'll be more confident and relaxed during the operation.

Some RK patients actually enjoy the operation. Very few enjoy the hours that follow, after the anesthetic has worn off! With RK, the "morning after" starts immediately, as we'll discover in our next chapter.

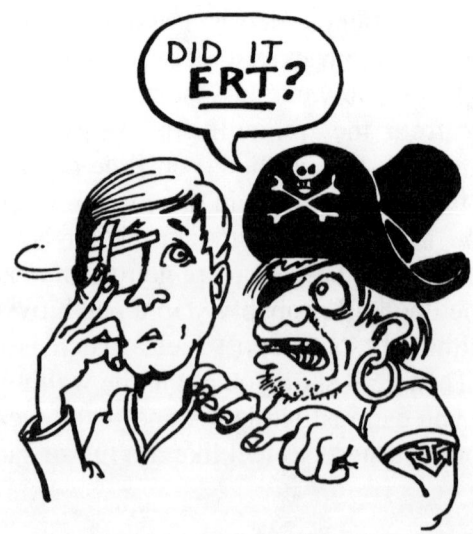

Sight For Sore Eye: The RK Recovery   10

You may feel pretty good as you relax on the ophthalmologist's couch after the operation, with your patched eye still numb and your brain still tranquil. It's hard to believe that within an hour you will be feeling positively awful, with a dull ache in your eye and a surly tone in your voice.

You are in for what ophthalmologists call "foreign body sensation": the feeling that something is in your eye, some foreign object no larger than a pineapple. You'll be given a prescription for a good painkiller, which you shouldn't take on an empty stomach. You probably will only need a few pills because this pain should be just about gone by the end of the following day.

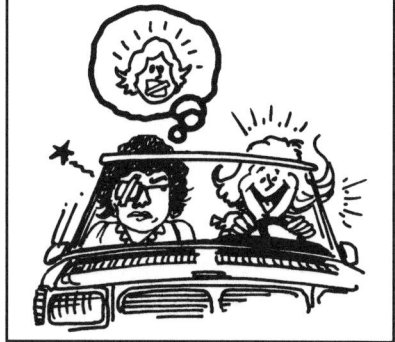

Day One

You'll be seeing the doc on the day after surgery, and probably also at one week, one month, three, six, and twelve months, and annually. The day-after meeting is vital to check for infection, but despite the sudden and exciting change in your vision, not much can be determined about the final result yet.

During the first days your vision may fluctuate every which way. RK is often over-effective at first, and then regresses; if this happens your vision may be farsighted for a week or two. While younger patients in this temporarily-overcorrected state may have 20/20 vision, those over forty may be unable to read through the operated eye for awhile. Don't assume you're overcorrected until the doctor says your eyes have probably stabilized.

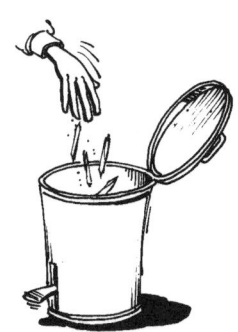

Remember: Using "Pot" may cause the operation to lose effect! Never use it during the recovery period if you don't want to see the RK result go up in smoke.

If you have both eyes done at one setting, as used to be common, the post-RK period can be nightmarish. You are led away blind, for starters, a Gothic-novel experience few of us care to sample. And when the patches are taken off, you may still find yourself blind except for the two-second glimpses for which you can force yourself to open one eye.

We'll assume for our discussion that you only have one eye operated on at a time!

When the patch comes off—nowadays most surgeons let you remove it a few hours after the operation—you will discover the meaning of the word *photophobia*, an incredible oversensitivity to light. If Francis Scott Key had been an RK patient, the dawn's early light would have sent him groping back to bed and we'd all be singing *Yankee Doodle* at ballgames.

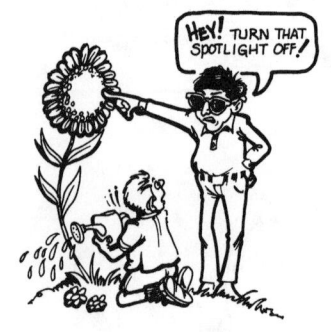

Gotta Wear Shades

I had to wear sunglasses for a month after the operation, especially in the mornings. To my amazement even the unoperated eye was light-sensitive, a touching display of fraternity. It can be a struggle to open your eyes in the morning, even in a moderately-bright room. It seems as if you and your eye are fighting for control of your eyelid, and your eye is both closer and meaner than you are so the lid stays closed.

The eye may also be watery, and the lid may be sore to the touch. You may be out of sorts as well from the painkillers. Don't try to drive.

Flare: a Star is Born

The other common minor complaint of recent RK patients is "flare", a starburst patterns around lights at night. This usually is quite noticeable in the weeks after surgery, and then diminishes. I noticed a tiny eight-pointed star around streetlights after my eight-incision RK surgery, and it is still with me almost three years later. Once every month or two I notice it, and can't help grinning. Of all the drawbacks and risks I was warned about, this is the worst that actually happened!

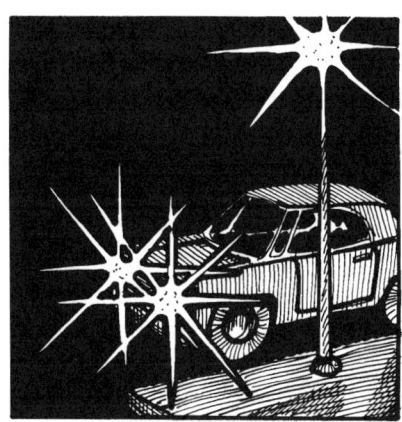

The star-patterns around lights at night are caused by the fact that the pupil dilates tremendously in the dark, to as much as sixteen times its daytime size (not so impressive, considering the eye is working with about one *ten-millionth* as much light). So the rays from the streetlights are going through a larger circle in the center of your cornea, including the inner ends of the RK scars. For the mildly-nearsighted patient with four or eight small scars around a big central clear zone, it will rarely be a problem, but for the higher myope with twelve or (Heaven forfend) sixteen scars closing in around a smaller optical zone, it may be significant. If you are a pilot or a truck driver with more than mild myopia, discuss this with your doctor.

Glare is a Bear

For some RK patients there is a related problem called "glare". This can occur at night or in the daytime, the cause being the diffusion of light as it strikes the RK incisions. Glare is a bright haze that makes vision less sharp and crisp, especially on sunny days. At its worst, glare makes the world look like you're viewing it through a screen door with the sun hitting it. About one fifth of RK patients are bothered by glare for the first couple of months, and then it usually goes away—in the meantime, dark glasses will handle the problem. This problem seems to be less common in recent years thanks to the better instruments being used; in fact many surgeons feel that RK causes less glare than contact lenses most of the time. Like the starbursts, glare is more likely to be significant for the more highly myopic patient.

You Look So Nice in the Evening, When I'm Nearsighted

Another frequent nuisance in the first month or two following RK, and sometimes longer, is fluctuating vision. The cornea following RK is somewhat flexible, so it can bulge or flatten as the forces on it change. You may have 20/20 vision in the morning, yet only 20/60 vision by evening because the eye becomes more nearsighted as the day passes. Very few patients have so much fluctuation that they wear different glasses in the morning and evening, but some do use glasses to drive home at night even though they don't need them on the way to work.

Normally this fluctuation, if it happens at all, will cease within a month or two. I never experienced this; it's more common in higher-myopia cases. But it could happen to you, and sometimes it can go on for as long as several years.

Steer Clear of Larry, Moe and Curly

Not only is it prone to slight fluctuations in curvature (and therefore focus), the incompletely-healed cornea also is more susceptible to injury. The danger is "blunt trauma", as ophthalmologists call a pop in the eye. Those unhealed incisions are weak—they have even less cohesion than the usual weakest point, the outer rim of the cornea.

Blunt trauma is a real threat to the RK'd eye. Just how much RK weakens the eye is controversial; a guesstimate would be that the eye is 50% less impact-resistant the day after the operation, and maybe 20% three months later. Probably after a year most corneas have healed well enough that the incisions are no longer the weak point, but it may be that for some patients at least, the eye remains slightly more fragile for three or four years, and possibly forever.

A Sense of What You Have to Lose

So protect that fresh RK operation! Wear eye protection in all projectile sports and contact sports. Stop fighting in bars (your mother and I really wish you would), avoid big excitable crowds, and generally be alert and aware of danger.

I no longer play hockey or handball, or even tennis, without eyewear—not so much because my RK'd eye may be slightly weaker than before, but because I used to take my eyes for granted, and now I don't. This may be true of anyone who undergoes any kind of eye surgery. If the RK experience gets the patient into the habit of guarding his eyes, one result of the operation may be that you make yourself be more careful.

One important tool for protecting your eyes is the seat belt. Example: a seventeen-year-old boy was in a head-on collision. Unbuckled, he hit the rear-view mirror and the frame of his glasses was mashed into his face. He was sadly certain that he'd lost an eye, but luck was with him. To this day I have a nice scar between my right eye and eyebrow as a reminder: wear your seatbelt!

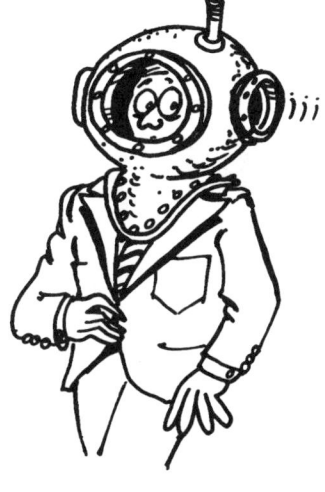

You don't have to go this far, but all RK alumni should buy some shop glasses to replace our prescription glasses during hobby hours.

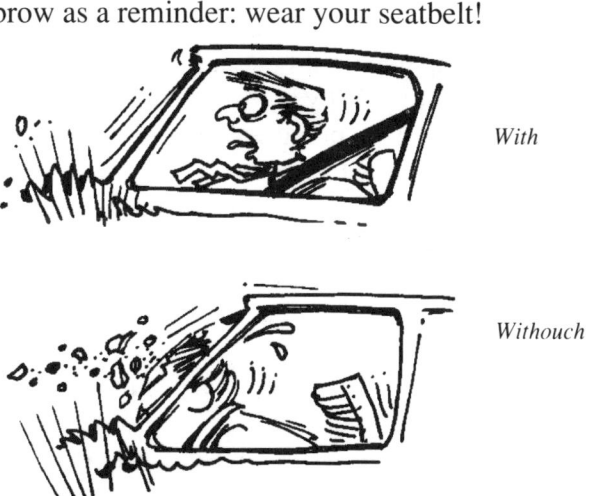

With

Withouch

Goggles for painting and handling chemicals, eyeguards for projectile sports, common sense, and an awareness of heightened danger can save your eyes whether you've had RK or not.

Don't Contaminate that RK

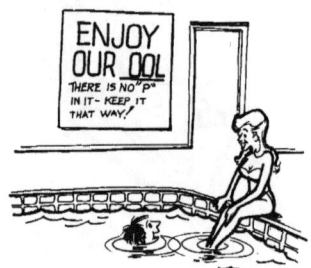

Immediately after the operation, the eye should be protected from soap and water, from chemicals and sources of infection such as are present in swimming pools, even in lakes or the ocean. A recent RK should not be exposed to dense cigarette smoke or to heavy industrial abuse such as dust, chemical mist or paint overspray.

What else should you know about the first month with RK? Well, some doctors will give you drops to use for several weeks, to guard against infection, or to aid in healing. Remember that the doctor can always spare a few minutes to see you if you have any unusual soreness, blurring, or any kind of problem or concern.

More "Thou-Shalt-Nots" for the Newborn RKaby

Your doc will advise you to try not to sleep on it, and may give you a little shield to wear over your RK'd eye at night. Avoid rubbing the eye excessively. Don't use mascara, eye shadow or any kind of makeup that could get in them, at least for the first week or so. Why take chances? Some surgeons may feel I'm being a worrywart with all these warnings, but what the heck—half the fun of surgery is making sacrifices you can gripe about.

You will probably be advised not to wear a contact lens in the operated eye for six to 12 months, because this can cause trouble. More on this later.

You may experience temporary "diplopia", or ghosting: a faint double image. This too will pass. And some people (non-monovision patients) are bothered by eye deviations during the period when only the first eye has been done, because the unoperated eye becomes "lazy". This stops when the second eye is done.

Your eyelid may be sore, and sometimes there's a small amount of ptosis—that's optho-talk for "droopy eyelid". Ptosis is not too pterrible, since it's almost always ptemporary.

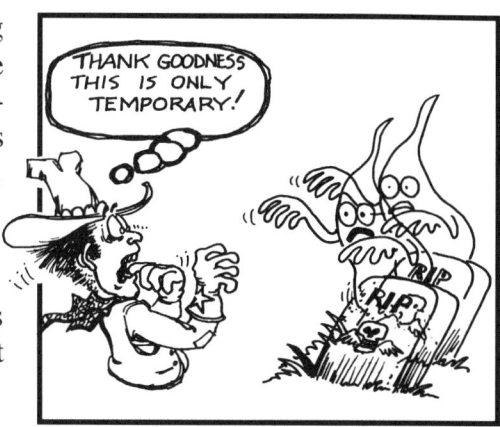

Right Between the Eyes: A Waiting Period

The person who gets both eyes done has two recovery periods. The second operation may be done as soon as six weeks after the first, or as long as a year or more; this should be completely up to the patient with the physician urging patience and caution every step of the way. A few surgeons like to operate on both eyes at once, which saves time and money, but prevents the result from the first eye being used to fine-tune the surgery in the second. Never allow this! In fact, the longer you wait before operating on the second eye, the better.

If you find that you have no problem with having only one corrected eye, you're a one-RK person. Stop right here! Three cheers for monovision! However, unless you are a one-eye tolerator, you probably will want to wear your glasses with a no-power lens over your RK'd eye. Of course, this causes a difference between the sizes of the image that the eyes receive, which sometimes results in headaches, especially if the diference between eyes is over four diopters. So a contact lens is better. If you can't tolerate a contact lens on the unoperated eye, you may find yourself very eager to get that second eye operated on. Try to be patient.

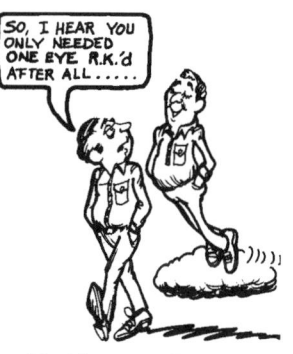

The Unexpected Monovisionary

Also go slow if your first eye seems to be undercorrected, and you want a re-operation to fine-tune it. Wait a few months to be sure the result has stabilized.

Caveat Eyeptor

The week after RK is a dangerous time for your operated eye. In addition to all the precautions we've described, be alert to any ominous developments. While watering and sticky lashes are normal, copious pus-production is not. If that thick yellow goo starts to flow, get down to your ophth's office pronto. That's a possible sign of infection. And while redness and soreness are standard, they should be getting better, not worse.

Be sure to use the antibiotic drops that the doc gives you. Wear an eye shield in bed if the doc thinks it's necessary. Don't miss any appointments, especially the first one.

Next: The Bottom Line

After your operation you probably won't be as concerned or excited about these various nuisances as you will be about the whole point of the enterprise—the results. How well will it work? If I still had my crystal ball I could tell you for sure, but how was I to know that little earthquake would knock it off the table? We'll have to settle for a look at the probabilities.

But Does It Work?
Results of RK

11

Immediately following the RK surgery, many patients' corneas "over-respond" to the operation, and flatten out more than desired. In the days and weeks that follow they unflatten somewhat, and usually stabilize within two months, although sometimes it takes longer, especially with the more highly myopic patients.

We've seen that the -2 D myope has better odds of success than the -6 D myope. In a minute, we'll look at the odds for each patient. First, a few general notes about RK outcomes.

There are three likely outcomes:

1. Perfection ("emmetropia", no error)

2. Undercorrection (still some myopia)

3. Over-correction (you've become farsighted, although if under 40 you may have 20/20 vision for now.)

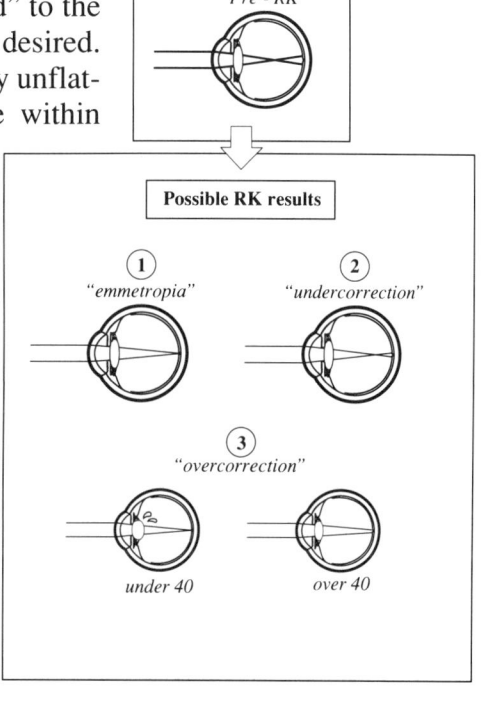

The ideal result, of course, is 20/20 or better, for life. However, since 20/40 is good enough for driving legally, and good enough that most people with 20/40 vision don't bother with glasses, this is usually considered the definition of RK success.

Outcome #2, undercorrection, is the commonest RK disappointment: the patient is still significantly nearsighted. If the patient plans to have both eyes operated, and the first eye comes out undercorrected, the surgeon will usually use a slightly stronger operation on the second eye, if possible. This should help improve the odds that the second eye comes out well and the patient is content.

Horseshoes and Hand Grenades

If the undercorrection is great enough to dissatisfy the patient, he may ask the surgeon to re-operate the still-myopic eye. Quite possibly this is feasible, and a second attempt will do the trick. They say that "close only counts in horseshoes and hand grenades", but it certainly counts in RK—and the RK practitioner can often pick 'er up and try another toss, which is not allowed with horseshoes nor recommended with hand grenades.

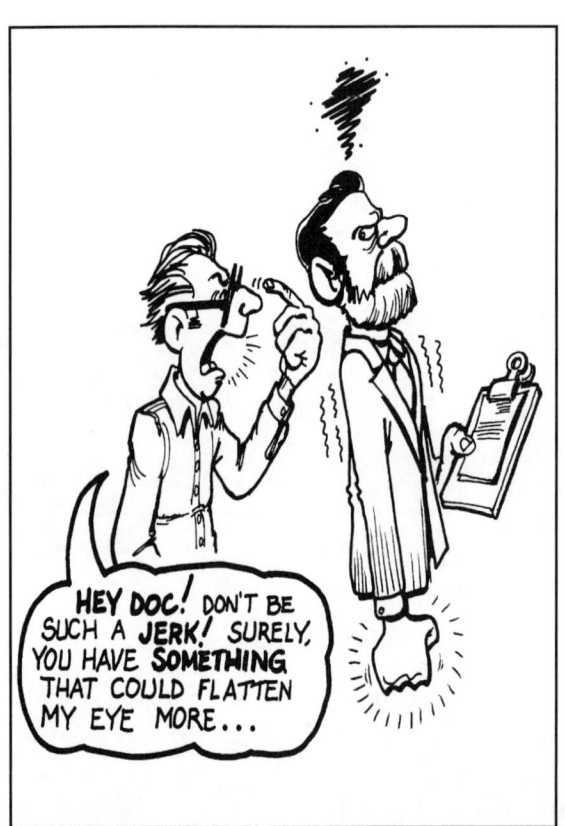

Sometimes that second operation is not likely to be successful, or is tried without producing much improvement. This is most likely to happen in the case of (you guessed it) the more highly-myopic patient, whose cornea may already be as flat as the doc can make it. If eight cuts with a 3mm optical clear zone still leave the eye undercorrected, re-operating even with eight more cuts is not likely to help. If such is the case, the patient will have to go back to glasses, although probably ones that are much thinner, less distorting—and easier to find!

One reason why it's important to accept in advance that the final result may not be 20/20 vision is the need to avoid pressuring the surgeon into repeated re-operation, which can lead to a permanently scarred cornea. Only one re-op should be tried, and that only if the surgeon believes it's likely to help.

When RK Works Too Well

Let's look at outcome #3. Over-correction, which is really over-response by the corneas of some patients, can be quite benign if you're just a kid (under 40, that is) and the hyperopia is minor, but it can be a bummer if you are over 40 and the overflattening is major. Until a technique of curing overcorrection is perfected it's important to be aware of this hazard.

In younger patients, the eye's ability to add power by accommodating often has the effect of sweeping overcorrection errors under the rug. Overcorrected RK patients, like other farsighted people, will start losing near vision earlier than others, and by sixty they won't even be able to see clearly in the distance. They'll probably wear bifocals, with a weak lens for distance and a stronger segment for reading.

Up to a diopter or so of overcorrection is not much trouble, especially if only one eye is RK'd and the other remains nearsighted for near vision. That's my own status: about one diopter overcorrected in my RK'd eye. I had a cycloplegic refraction done recently, so that with paralyzed accommodation I could see the kind of vision I'll have in my presbyopic years. It wasn't 20/20 but it was not too bad, not blurry enough to bother with glasses except maybe for driving.

People who get both eyes overcorrected are the unhappiest patients. We myopes make unhappy hyperopes! It's jarring to discover that no matter how close you hold your watch, you still can't read it. Additional RK can't help; re-operating would only make the hyperopia worse.

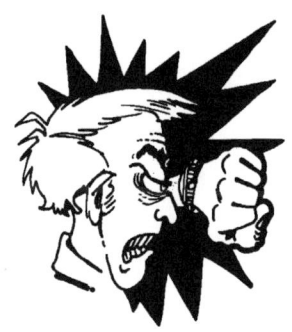

Double-barreled overcorrection can usually be prevented by the conservative approach to RK: the lean-toward-undercorrection strategy, with enough of a wait between operations to be sure your first eye is not overcorrected. Once he's aware of the first eye's overresponse, the surgeon can use a less powerful operation on the second eye and usually prevent the same thing from happening there.

RK for the Mild, Moderate and Major Myopes

In studying the probable results, RK could be viewed as three distinct operations, because the prospects are so different for low myopia (one to three diopters), moderate myopia (three to six diopters) and high myopia (six to ten diopters).

The mildly nearsighted person has the best prospects. For starters, he or she may be able to have only one eye corrected, and be perfectly happy with the result: a dominant eye with keen distance vision, and the non-dominant eye left nearsighted for reading and close vision in the presbyopic decades. This means half the cost, half the recovery nuisances, half of all the remote risks, and a certainty of retaining that one blessing of myopia—near vision in middle and senior years. Built-in bifocals!

Low Myopia = High Odds of Success

The mildly myopic individual has around a 60% chance of coming away with 20/20 vision or better, and about a 90% chance of 20/40 or better—good enough to drive legally, perhaps wearing glasses to drive at night. (The mildest myopes, in the -1 to -2D range, often do much better: in one published series of 86 very-low patients, 100% obtained 20/20!) RK is also more trouble-free for the low myopes—the big uncut optical zones tend to minimize the side effects and the chances of any complication, as we'll see in the next chapter.

It is a paradox that the low myope is the most likely to come away from RK with excellent vision, but is also the least motivated to seek RK.

Moderately Good Odds

For the moderate, -3 D to -6 D myope, the odds are slightly less inviting—depending where in this range one falls (I must admit that although I'm a -3.5 D, I tend to group myself with the low myopes. The -3D cut-off point is pretty arbitrary; it's really a continuum, not three distinct clusters.) Most patients over -3D will want both eyes done, although some people can handle up to five diopters of mismatch between their eyes. Even if you do want both eyes done, you should do some testing to see if the second eye can be half-corrected, to retain "presbyopia insurance".

As the degree of unwanted myopia increases, so does the likelihood of missing the bullseye and coming away with imperfect vision. Undercorrection can still sometimes be fixed by reoperation, but not as often as with low myopia.

The -4 or -5 D moderate myope has about an 80% chance of achieving 20/40 vision, and about a 50% chance of 20/20. Of course, some of the 20/20 patients will be mildly overcorrected patients, and will eventually find themselves farsighted—this may be something like 10% of them.

Still, these odds are attractive to people who strongly dislike the eyewear alternatives, and even those who get less than 20/40 are usually better off than before. For example, they probably can read or watch television comfortably without glasses.

A Testimonial

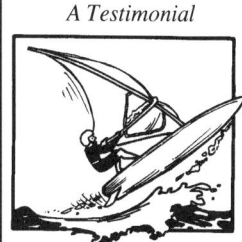

"When my mast broke while windsurfing Turnagain Arm, Alaska, in July of 1988, John spotted me in the water from about a mile away and sailed out with a towline. So this RK stuff must work at least some of the time! I'm for it.

- J.S., Anchorage, AK

High Myopia: Lower Expectations

For high myopia, above six or seven diopters, the odds against getting enough correction from RK to give you 20/20 or even 20/40 get pretty steep, and age becomes a major factor. Nowadays most surgeons will use RK on highly myopic patients only if they're at least middle-aged, and/or promise to be happy with an undercorrection. For the younger hi-my patient, the chances of 20/40 are less than 50—50! The likelihood of 20/20 is maybe one chance in five. We'll look at this complex picture closely in the chapter after next.

Any significant degree of astigmatism lowers the probability of complete success. If you have two or three diopters of astigmatism, you should lower the probability of 20/20 by 15 percentage points, and lower the probability of 20/40 by at least ten points. More than three diopters of astigmatism mean you need to read chapter 15.

Wanted: a Better RK Yardstick

As the years pass, and more doctors specialize in RK and compile their results, there will come to be a standardized method of reporting results. It is a surprisingly tricky problem: just how do you measure RK results?

What is success? The usual standard is "20/40 or better", which tells us nothing about overcorrection—in a 30-year-old patient, a significant overcorrection could be hidden by the patient's accommodation, leaving him with hawkeyed 20/15 for the time being. So when you read "90% chance of 20/40 or better", remember that some of those 90% of happy people will eventually be farsighted.

The Plus-or-Minus One Diopter Standard

Another common standard is the percentage of patients who come away "within plus-or-minus one diopter of emmetropia"—that is, with no more than one D of myopia or of hyperopia, whether they have perfect vision or not. This yardstick doesn't allow the patient's accommodation to conceal future hyperopia. But what does it tell us? How good is "within one diopter"?

Take that +1 D outcome, that is, overcorrected by one diopter. How much trouble is a diopter of latent farsightedness, which won't even rear its ugly head until you're 40? Again, if you're twenty-five and only having one eye operated on, it's nothing to lose sleep over—you've got fifteen or twenty years of perfect distance vision coming, and lifelong near vision with your other eye. But if you're forty-five and both eyes are overcorrected by one diopter, you may feel that you're more glasses-dependent than before. Obviously, no surgeon wants to overcorrect both eyes, especially with a 45-year-old patient—most surgeons are especially cautious about overcorrecting presbyopic patients. But you can see that the nuisance value of a mild hyperopic result varies acording to the circumstances.

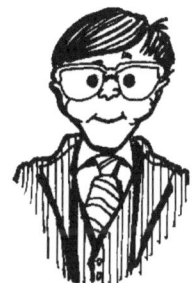 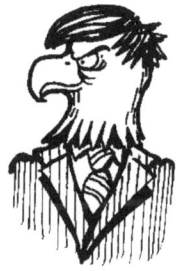 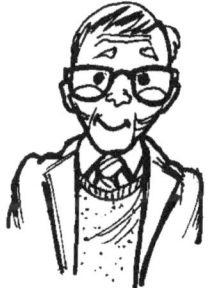

Portrait of the Myope as a young man.   *After **overcorrecting** RK he may have 20/20 or better for years.*   *By age 40, needs bifocals—can't see far or near unaided.*

The Devil You Know

Undercorrection is more familiar: you're still a little nearsighted. Very few RK patients remain even half as nearsighted as before the operation—even undercorrected patients are much improved. And the passing years only make the remnant myopia more desirable, for its near-vision advantages. Still, even going from 20/400 to 20/60 can be a disappointment for some people.

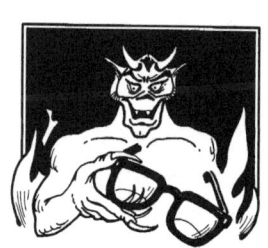

*It's not really **this** bad!*

What kind of vision do you have if you're one diopter undercorrected? Anywhere from 20/20 to 20/60, it seems. The cornea is never exactly spherical, and after RK it's even less so—many RK'd patients have much better vision than their refractions would suggest.

So, the "+/- 1 diopter of emmetropia" guage is pretty nebulous, except to say that the vast majority of patients within those bounds will be delighted with their result, and so will many patients outside those bounds. The young monovisionary with 1.5 D of hidden hyperopia (farsightedness) in his operated eye will be clicking his heels for the next twenty years every time he thinks of his vision, and the formerly -6 D myope who couldn't read without glasses, and comes out -1.5 D and needs them only for night driving, will break into fits of uncontrolled grinning for years before she starts taking it for granted.

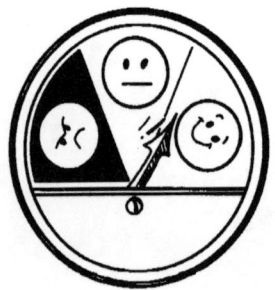

The Happometer Chart

One way to report results would be a simple happiness chart, which might look like this. The figures are my own guesstimates, based on all the results I am aware of.

Degree of Pre-op myopia	less than 2D	2 to 4D	4 to 6D	6 to 8D	above 8D
% happy with results after one year	95%	90%	85%	80%	75%
% likely to still be happy at age 50	95%	85%	75%	80%	75%
% really disappointed	1%	5%	10%	10%	20%

That's my best shot. It reflects the fact that presbyopia will decrease the percentage of happy patients slightly. Many ophthalmologists will take issue, especially with the low figure for high-myope happiness, because they screen such patients rigorously and only accept those who don't demand a full correction to be satisfied. In fact, many of the most deliriously overjoyed patients are ex-high myopes who become ordinary low myopes after RK! Dr. Salz of Los Angeles, for example, does not perform RK on higher-myopia patients unless they're older, and willing to accept a -2 D or -3 D result, and finds 90% of them are happy.

Good Odds, No Guarantees

To summarize, no patient has a "sure thing" with RK, but the odds of getting at least 20/40 are very good for the mild myope (especially if he or she is also a monovision candidate), not quite as good for the moderate myope, and rather poor for the high myope or the astigmatic person. Yet for the right person in any category, RK can be great. Your chances of being pleased probably depend to a large degree on how hard-to-please you are, as well as on your pre-operative vision.

The outcome may also be affected by your post-operative activity. Smoking pot, we've noted, lowers the intraocular pressure and may cause an undercorrection (or, theoretically, may reduce an overcorrection). Dr. Michael Deitz suspects that patients who spend time outdoors get more effect than those who read all day. Some say that weight-lifters get unpredictable results. As time passes, such patterns will become clearer.

Next, let's take a look at the remarkable RK decision, particularly as confronted by low and moderate myopes. Then we'll have chapters for the higher myopes and astigmatic folks, and a look at choosing your surgeon, paying for RK, and the Future.

Potential Problems with RK 12

Only human beings, at least within four light years of here, ever have to painstakingly weigh the value of a benefit against a possible danger. Animals can't really do it, and presumably God doesn't have to—as usual, we humans are at that awkward in-between stage.

We Can't be Descended from Apes— They're Too Intelligent

We're not very good at it. Half of us don't use a seat belt, for example, even though any benefits of skipping the buckle-up hardly weigh against the ghastly risks of not wearing it. And we rarely consider the risks we take with our eyes. When we set off firecrackers, work with power tools, pour corrosive chemicals or play raquetball, nobody is standing there telling us that we are taking such-and-such a chance of blinding an eye.

All surgery has hazards, even relatively minor surgery. The currently fashionable thigh-fat suctioning operation, for example, has actually killed eleven patients! RK is among the least risky of all eye surgeries, and certainly hasn't killed anybody, but it is surgery and does entail some risk. Your ophthalmologist will tell you so, and ask that you confirm your awareness of the risk—in writing. You may feel that the hazards are acceptable considering the probable benefits, but you must be aware of the worst that could happen.

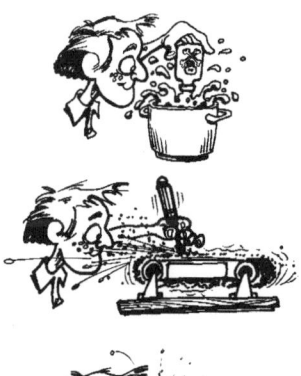

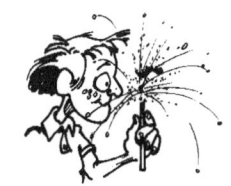

This guy won't read this chapter

I'll try to present the risks with some sense of proportion, but it isn't easy. With about 250,000 patients, probably everything that can go wrong has, and it's a fairly long list. I may have missed one or more risks, so *be sure to listen closely to your surgeon and ask him about possible problems.*

Sudden Vision

> *It's impossible to be sure you have listed all the possible complications! We may have missed one, so ask your ophthalmologist. He's the final authority.*

RK today is safer than it was as recently as five years ago, and many good surgeons have never seen a serious complication. Hopefully, few of my readers will have cause to regret RK. Still, it's a fact: some patients do regret RK.

The Worst that Could Happen

Nobody has ever been completely blinded because of RK, but about a dozen patients have lost sight in one eye. About half of these disasters were caused by injections of anesthetic that damaged the optic nerve; since injected anesthetic is rarely used for RK any more we won't dwell on that hazard.

The two most serious RK threats are infection and blunt trauma.

A major infection inside the eye is the worst thing that can happen to any eye-surgery patient. This nightmare has a name: endophthalmitis. It can sometimes be cured with antibiotics, but when this fails the retina is likely to be damaged and vision in the infected eye may be lost.

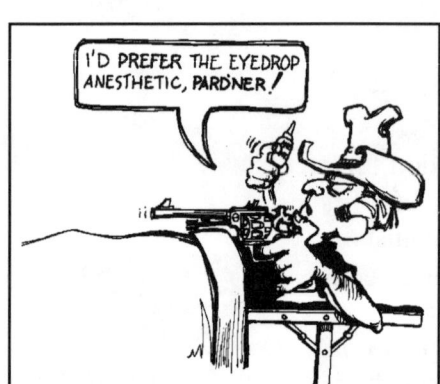

Patient expressing opinion on choice of anesthetic.

Since RK incisions normally do not penetrate the inner layers of the cornea, there is normally no possibility of such an infection. However, as we have seen, tiny perforations do occur in about 5% of all operations, especially high-myopia cases where maximum-depth incisions are used. Such perforations can provide an opportunity for microbes to enter the eye. It seems that they do so, and start an infection, in about one out of fifteen or twenty thousand RK patients.

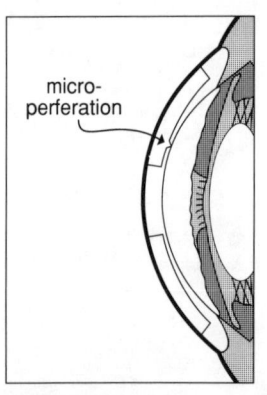

A microperforation: cause for carefulness, not alarm

Post-Perf Precautions

Endophthalmitis is much more common in cataract surgery, in which the clouded lens is removed. With RK such an infection is twenty times less likely, and also easier to cure because the lens is still there and may block the infection's spread to the back of the eye.

Make sure your surgeon alerts you if there's a microperforation in your surgery. These tiny punctures—unlike larger "macroperforations", which force the doc to stop the operation and finish it several weeks later—are so minor a problem that the doc may never even mention it unless you ask him to in advance. Although the chance of infection is small—perhaps one in a thousand—you can make it even smaller by avoiding contamination, and contacting the surgeon immediately if you suspect trouble.

Another very rare complication (probably more common with contacts than with RK) is an infection of the cornea itself, bacterial keratitis. This almost always clears up fast with treatment. If your cornea suddenly seems to be having problems, don't be shy about bothering your ophthalmologist on his day off. Once in a great while serious damage to the cornea can occur. Be particularly alert if you wear a contact lens after RK; check your corneas daily in the mirror. This is one complication that can develop weeks or months—even years— after the surgery.

A Cautionary Tale

We've already mentioned the other way that RK can result in tragic loss: blunt trauma, a hard blow to the operated eye. There have been a small number of such cases, including serious auto accidents as well as fistfights. Just how weak the eye is depends on how recent the operation, how many incisions, possibly the age of the patient (younger patients seem to heal faster) and so on. Sometimes the post-RK cornea holds up better than you might expect: an RK'd pilot who crashed his plane in the Rocky Mountains suffered fractures of the facial bones around the eyes, yet the RK incisions held.

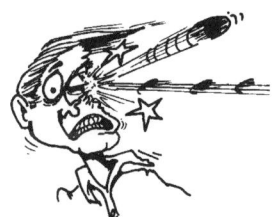

Wear protection! Even plastic sunglasses are better than nothing.

And here's a case of a man who took a flying raquetball in his eye just a few days after the operation. Yowch! Although it hurt plenty, the cornea held and no permanent damage was done. Has a patron saint of Radial Keratotomy already been appointed?

Assuming that you have a competent surgeon and that no injected anesthetic is used, infection and hard impact are the two things that could actually blind an eye. There is perhaps one chance in twenty thousand that one of these things will happen to you, odds that would be more frightening if we had only one eye apiece—in fact, RK is never performed on patients with only one good eye, and most surgeons believe both eyes should never be RK'd at the same time. Even the most remote risk of blinding one eye is a serious matter and should discourage anyone who is not really unhappy with glasses or contacts.

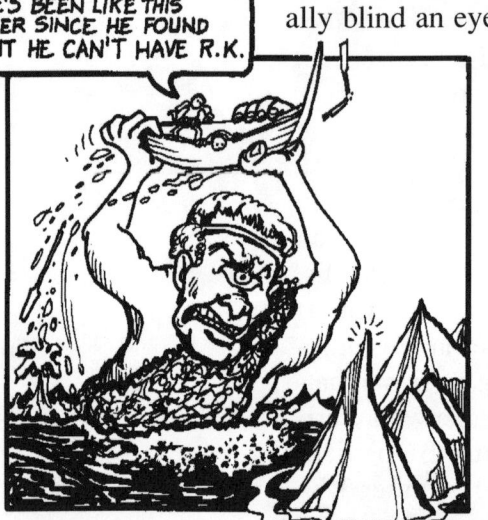

Less Frightful but More Likely

There's more. In fact, more people may be discouraged by the list of less serious, but more likely pitfalls that we will examine next.

The most likely misfortune, of course, is imperfect correction: too much or too little. We've dealt with these already. We'll discuss them further in the next chapter on the RK decision.

We've already discussed the problem of glare, in which "crispness" of vision is decreased. This rarely becomes a permanent nuisance, but once in awhile it may—usually in cases of higher myopia. Sometimes a sudden head-jerk by the patient causes a sloppy incision that results in some degree of permanent glare.

Some patients report decreased night vision. These are usually patients with some residual myopia. At night the pupil opens wide, and the less-corrected outer part of the cornea gets into the picture. Glasses can be prescribed for night driving; the testing for this prescription should be done in a dark room, with only the chart illuminated.

Fluctuating vision is a problem we've mentioned—a tendency for the cornea to become more rounded as the day progresses, making you more nearsighted toward evening. Usually the change is half a diopter or less—very rarely enough to require the use of two pairs of glasses.

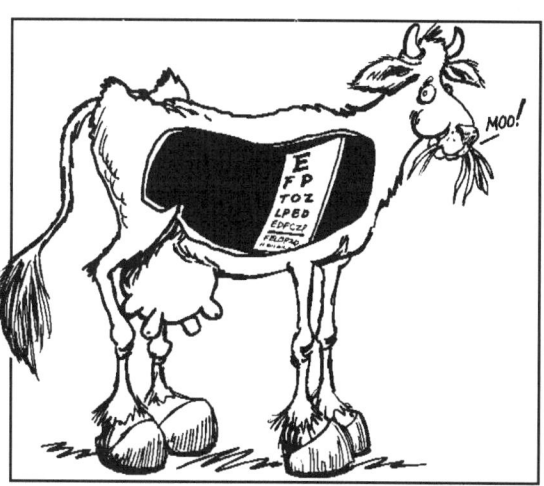

As we say down home, "darker'n the inside of a cow"

Normally this fluctuation, if it happens, will cease within a month or two, but sometimes it can go on for several years, perhaps longer. It used to be thought that the cornea could not take so long to stabilize, but the PERK study has shown long-term fluctuating vision in a significant minority of patients. Again the problem is much more likely to be serious for the highly-myopic patient whose surgeon used deeper incisions; some experts speculate that the deep incisions leave too much flexibility in the cornea and make fluctuating vision more likely.

"But I Thought That Was What You Wanted", said the Cornea

Vision after RK can also fluctuate in a different way: the eye can continue to become slightly less nearsighted, or more farsighted, for several years. A patient who had 20/20 after the operation might be farsighted two years later. The same phenomenon causes some undercorrected patients to find their vision continuing to get better, with less and less nearsightedness as the months go by. It may be that deep incisions, such as are used when maximum effect is needed, cause some corneas to keep on flattening long after the operation—as if, after decades of stubborn inflexibility, they just can't stop trying to be helpful.

Fortunately, these long-term fluctuations are usually mild—a total change of one or two diopters or less. Since nearsighted people often experience slight shifts in their refractions, it may turn out that the eye is partly to blame. And the excessively-deep incisions of the early 80's may be implicated. There is considerable speculation about this as our book goes to press; as in other areas, your doctor will be able to fill you in on more recent findings.

Occasionally the RK operation causes astigmatism. This is uncommon, and more likely to happen in the highly-myopic cases. Mild astigmatism of one diopter or less is not usually noticeable, but occasionally more than that is caused. If this "induced astigmatism" is irregular in nature, it can be very difficult to correct—only a gas-permeable rigid (GPR) contact lens works well in some cases.

Double Vision in a Single Eye

Some patients, again usually high-myopia ones, experience a ghostly double-image. This usually is temporary, but can be permanent if caused by irregular induced astigmatism. This is rare, but it happens—two of the 435 PERK study patients were troubled by double vision.

There may be other types of mild distortion or ghosting which result in the patient's "best corrected vision" being less than it was before the operation. After all, before the operation nearly all patients have excellent vision with their glasses or contacts on, at least as far as the Snellen chart can measure it. After the operation, vision is almost certain to be much better than unaided vision before the operation, but any minor irregularity caused by the incisions may cause vision to be slightly imperfect, and thus less than the preoperative glasses-on vision.

Depends on How You Look At It

The possibility that the patient's best-corrected vision may decrease after RK has been used to attack the operation. However, this is a subjective problem—consider the case of the -6 D myope who could read the 20/20 line with his glasses on before RK. Suppose that after the RK he has 20/60 vision, and even with new glasses he still has only 20/30. Technically, he has "lost two Snellen lines of best-corrected acuity" and will be considered evidence of RK's failings. But if you ask him, he may tell you that his vision is now undistorted— squares are no longer barrel-shaped—plus he gets a full-sized rather than a shrunken image, has wide peripheral vision for the first time, and no longer feels helpless without glasses.

In some cases, however, the decrease in best-corrected vision is more significant, so this has to be considered as a potential drawback.

Ouch

There may be temporary erosions of the corneal epithelium—scratchy spots where the epithelium rubs off. These can be cured with eyedrops that lubricate the cornea. This used to be more common in the days of relatively crude steel knives; the new diamond blades don't tear up the epithelium much at all.

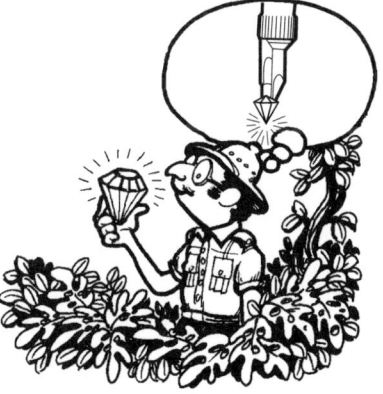

Dear Ann Landers: My Husband has a Wandering Eye

If you ever had a problem with one eye being "weak" and having a tendency to turn inward or outward, it is possible that RK may aggravate this problem, especially during the period when only one eye has been done, when you are waiting to have the second eye RK'd. When the second eye is done, the deviation usually disappears. One study showed this problem in one out of three hundred patients.

The Post-RK Fitting Problem: Baron von Contact's Revenge

One legacy of RK is the contact lens problem. Contacts should not be worn at all for several months after RK—tiny capillaries may grow into the cornea from the perimeter if lenses are used too soon, especially soft ones. Even after this danger has passed, it can be difficult to satisfactorily fit contact lenses on the RK'd eye.

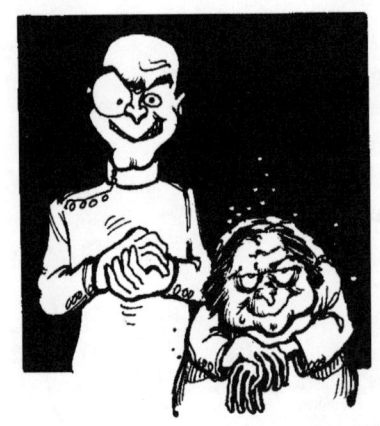

Of course, many RK patients could not tolerate contacts to begin with, which was why they wanted RK. If all goes well, contacts won't be needed after the operation. As we've seen, however, some patients get too little or too much correction. Especially if there is an uncomfortable difference between the two eyes, the RK patient may turn to contact lenses.

Generally, the less effective the operation the easier it is to fit contacts afterward. Overcorrected patients whose corneas have been markedly flattened are the hardest to fit satisfactorily.

Contact lens technology continues to advance, and as there come to be more ex-RK patients around, the contact engineers are developing new lenses that can be worn on flattened corneas. And already some ophthalmologists, optometrists and opticians are getting much better at helping RK patients; many of the high-volume RK surgeons know such a professional. The new rigid gas-permeable lenses are often the best bet, while extended-wear softies are the worst. Nevertheless, if you can wear contacts comfortably now, you should be aware that you may not be able to do so after the surgery.

We've mentioned microperforations. Sometimes a larger perforation occurs, when the surgeon unwittingly cuts a line a millimeter or two in length through the cornea. Usually this "macroperforation" will be closed with a tiny stitch, and the operation will be halted, and completed a week or two later when the macroperforation has healed. Usually no permanent harm is done, but observe the precautions we outlined for microperforations.

RK and the Endothelium

One other long-range fear that has worried some ophthalmologists is the possibility of damage to the endothelium, that fragile single layer of cells that seals the cornea off from the aqueous fluid inside the eye. Many studies have been done to learn how many of these cells die off after RK; results run from 2% to 7%. Re-operation of the same eye probably has an equal kill-rate. Long experience with other types of eye surgery—most of them more violent to the cornea, such as cataract surgery, which involves a large incision at the limbus—suggest that this much damage to the endothelium will have no ill effect. Some experts say that contact lenses probably cause more damage to the endothelium than RK. As the years pass, fear of RK endothelium damage seems to be di-

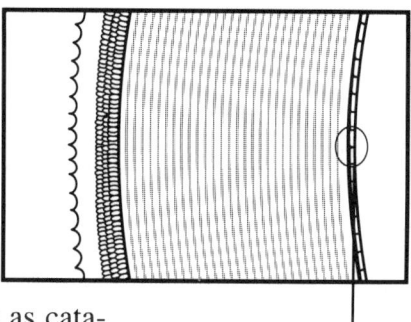

Endothelium

minishing.

There have been a few really rare misfortunes. A few patients have developed cataracts (lens clouding), usually due to prolonged post-operative steroid use. Once the epithelium grew down through an incision; that was treated successfully. And at least once, the retina was damaged by the operating light during an unusually long RK, prompting surgeons to be more cautious about minimizing the brightness and duration of light.

That pretty well covers the risks, unless you count the jaw ache from constant grinning for three weeks after the operation, or the hazard of violence at the hands of nearsighted friends who lose patience with your smug expression. Seriously, most risks can be lowered if the patient follows his doctor's instructions and the precautions outlined in the previous chapter.

Talk to your surgeon about all of these potential problems, read the literature he gives you and question him closely. You and your surgeon will have to live with the results, not I, so don't take my word for gospel in this. Make sure that you understand the risks before you go through with it.

RK versus the Contact Lens

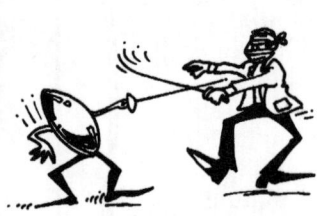

The debate goes on as to whether RK is more dangerous than contacts. It's hard to say, since the RK risk is basically a one-shot affair, whereas the risks with contacts are continuous—corneal ulcers, infection or giant papillary conjunctivitis (GPC) can strike any time you get lazy or careless with your disinfecting or cleaning. Induced astigmatism can be caused by contacts, and long-term damage to the endothelium may occur. Even glasses cause plenty of lost eyes every year due to shattering, although they also protect many people from chemical splashes and projectiles.

Writing this chapter got me so interested in eye

Potential Problems

risks that I also researched and wrote several pages on various eye hazards and eye first aid—please read the last chapter, "Eyemergencies". And for you contacteers, there's a whole chapter on those little devils.

Most professionals still believe that contacts are less hazardous than RK. It may be true that a larger percentage of contact wearers than RK patients will eventually develop some problem significant enough to cause a doctor's visit, but the great majority will be easily treatable. RK is more likely than contacts to cause a permanent new visual flaw, usually mild farsightedness (overcorrection), which probably occurs about 5% to 10% of the time.

RK's major drawback is also its great advantage: it's permanent. You don't have to put it in every morning or buy a new pair twice a year, but by the same token it's hard to adjust if imperfect, or if your eyesight changes.

Contact-lens disasters are often the patient's fault, and self-inflicted contact nightmares may become even more common if extended-wear lenses from volume outlets replace well-supervised daily wear, so be wary.

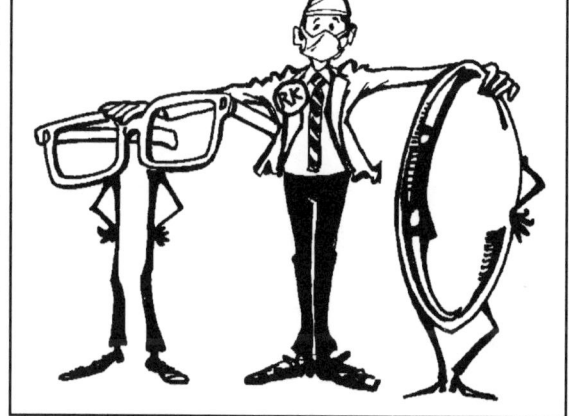

Basically, glasses are for all that can be happy with them. Contacts are for those who can tolerate and care for them, and hate glasses. RK is for those who despise both of the older solutions, and are willing to accept RK's possible risks and shortcomings. Each of the three is the right choice for some people. Certainly RK is safer than going around with blurry vision, as some people do.

Which is the right choice for you? In our next chapter, let's take a look at the RK Decision.

The RK Decision   13

It's Great to Have a Choice!

"Should I give RK a shot, and try to do something about my nearsightedness?"

What a remarkable option. It's a decision unlike any we've faced before, and so new that few of us can be advised by friends who have been there. Instead, we are the ones others will turn to for guidance in years to come.

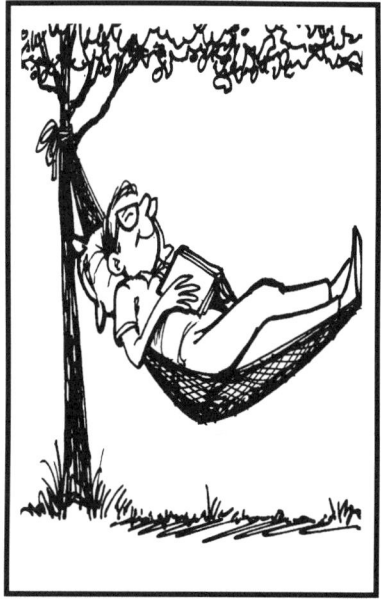

We've now explored the whole RK landscape, including the recovery, the probabilities for success, and the various dangers and drawbacks. We have seen that the prospects vary according to how nearsighted (and astigmatic) you are to start with. The low myope has the best odds, and possibly only needs one eye done. The moderate nearseer gets slightly worse odds and usually wants both eyes done—hopefully, one eye can be left mildly nearsighted. The highly myopic person has a more complex decision to make, has other operations to consider, and has a whole 'nother chapter to read after this one.

Come Back after Your Eye Exam

Of course, you can't make the decision until after you've had the pre-RK exam and talked it over with your surgeon. You'll find out how good a candidate you are and whether there are any "contra-indications", and ask all the questions this book has left you with. Then you can come back and re-read this chapter, which is just a grab-bag of thoughts and ideas that may be of help. The decision, of course, is yours to make, and please don't go either way because of anything I tell you. I'm just trying to be helpful, not to "steer" you.

Either Way You Look at It, You Win

Any decision is likely to be a good one if it is executed wisely. If you decide to go ahead with RK, this means you should start by accepting that you may *not* be completely freed from glasses. It means carefully choosing a doctor to do your surgery and following all instructions, including possible sacrifices such as giving up contact sports, eye shadow or marijuana for a while. You'll have to do your part before, during, and after the operation.

If you decide to "pass" on RK or to wait a few more years, doing *that* right means taking good care of your eyes for the rest of your life—how else can you get your money's worth out of this book? Don't miss Appendices B and C on Contacts and Eyemergencies. If still interested in eventually using RK or another refractive procedure to upgrade your vision, you should monitor future developments as suggested in Chapter 17.

And please, be generous! Can you imagine how it would feel to be stuck waiting for a clear cornea transplant? Fill out the Eye Bank donor form in Appendix C, and stick it in your wallet.

The Big Two and the Others

When deliberating RK—assuming the doctor has determined that you're a good candidate—you have two major factors to consider and many minor ones. The Big Two: how nearsighted you are, and how badly you want not to be. We've certainly looked at #1, and #2 is your department. So let's take a look at some of the other factors.

Can you tolerate "monovision", and make do with only one eye corrected? If so, the whole hassle is cut right down to half-size, and bare-eyed near vision is preserved for later years.

If you do need both eyes done, can you tolerate having one eye only partially corrected? If so, then even though you'll need both eyes operated upon, at least you can avoid reading glasses in presbyopia-time.

Your age affects the decision in several ways. The non-monovision candidate, who will need both eyes fully corrected, will be more enthusiastic if he's twenty, and has 25 years before presbyopia, than if he's forty and will soon need reading glasses if he undergoes RK. For the monovision candidate this is not a factor—in fact, monovision's potential escape-route from bifocals may make RK even more attractive to the older person. For highly myopic individuals too, RK grows more attractive in their 40's and 50's because a much greater correction can be achieved.

> Over-40 patients should make sure the surgeon operates on the cautious side. Overcorrection is worse if you're presbyopic!

Can you afford it? RK may be covered under your insurance or it may not. See Chapter 16 for insurance pointers and a bunch of ideas on paying for it.

Can You Handle Disappointment?

Are you accustomed to situations in which the outcome is not predictable? Some people are angry and bitter if things don't happen to turn out perfectly, while others shrug it off and get on with life. If you are an anxious, demanding person, RK is probably not a good idea for you. Many ophthalmologists say that engineers, attorneys and accountants are particularly likely to be miserable if the result is not a perfect 20/20; don't know why that would be. For some people (in any profession) it's hard to accept that they can have a setback without it being somebody's fault.

It has been said that only a few percent of RK patients are really unhappy, but those few are *really* unhappy. It seems that the patients with considerable astigmatism as well as myopia are often the ones who end up deeply disappointed.

Eagles and Owls

It's fair to ask whether RK will advance your career. For a lifeguard, pilot, security guard, model, actor, dancer, salesman, executive, or athlete the answer *may* be yes.

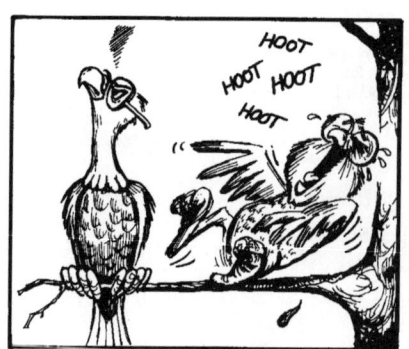

Tens of thousands of people have been able to enter demanding professions like firefighting, paramedic, and police thanks to RK. (But be sure to check with such prospective employers in advance. Incredibly, some exclude RK alumni from employment. That's unreasonable discrimination.)

On the other hand, some young executives feel that glasses make them look older (and wiser?) than they really are; if so they could be in trouble if the truth gets out. It seems that people with glasses are stereotyped as more intelligent and trustworthy; without them they are seen as more attractive and successful. What do you do if in your work you need to appear both intelligent *and* successful? Wear a monocle?

Should You Give Contacts Another Try?

Although some feel otherwise, the consensus is still that contacts are safer than RK, and many surgeons will ask whether you've given the recent generations of contacts a chance. Remember: you have to follow instructions with contacts, or you will run into trouble eventually. Read Appendix B! And make sure you've got a good professional; the fast-service, high-volume outfits rarely provide the personal care you want with contacts.

There is some truth to this rule: The glasses-hater who hasn't tried contacts is not yet a likely RK candidate. The miserable contact-wearer or contact non-tolerator *may* be, and the most likely candidate of all is the person who lives with poor vision rather than wear glasses or contacts. For such people, RK may be safer than no RK.

RK and the Army, Part One

Don't have RK so you can join the armed forces. This is (as I write, and hopefully as you read) peacetime, with no draft, and it's easy to be ineligible to serve your country. Have you had a minor bowel obstruction in the past five years? You're out. It's the same with RK: for the present, the U.S. Armed Services will not induct RK'd applicants. Dr. Kramer, advisor for Ophthalmology to the Surgeon General of the Army, told me that while RK results so far look good, the Army will wait a little longer—possibly a complete review in 1990 or thereabouts. "We're only concerned about resistance to blunt trauma, which is still uncertain, and other long-term health considerations," he explains. "Undercorrection and overcorrection are no problem for us, since we're only looking at the people who've passed our vision test already."

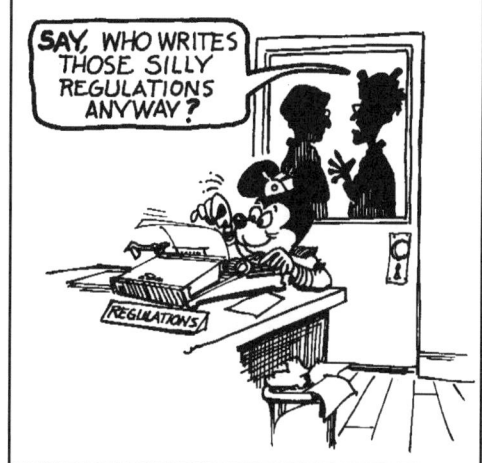

He pointed out that the Army's policy could change quickly in the event of war. So let's hope it changes slowly! It certainly should change, because it is pretty clear that the added liability, or risk of battlefield incapacity, that the Army assumes with an RK'd soldier is absurdly small, compared to the benefit such a motivated, self-improving enlistee is likely to bring to his country's service. (In the Army's defense, it has set up its own RK service in Colorado, free to all military dependents and retirees. See Chapter 16.)

Highly-myopic long-haul truck drivers and others who need excellent night vision may shy away from RK, since the starburst may annoy them too much—especially if they get undercorrected, and still need glasses. Between the star effects and the reflections off your glasses, the view could get cluttered.

Projectile Sports can Impact Your Decision

If you are hoping to be able to play at sports without eyewear after RK, remember that the RK'd eye may be more susceptible to severe injury from "blunt trauma". If you have been envious of your handball buddy who plays with nothing over his eyes, stop being jealous of his eyepower and start being concerned about his brainpower. Everyone should wear eye protection for such high-impact activities, especially after RK.

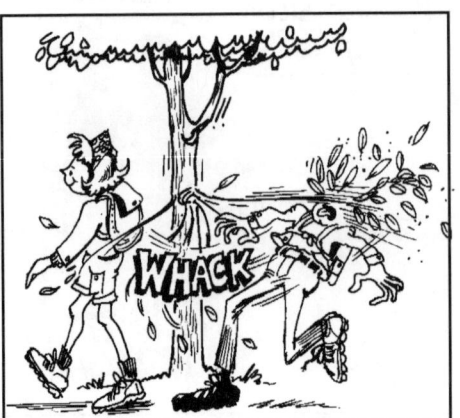

The Author's own Post-RK close call

Lifestyle affects the decision, of course—for instance, how much of your activity is physical and how much is mental. If your days are spent hoisting crabpots in the Bering Sea (sounds unlikely, but my neighbor does that for a living) then you may be more excited about RK than if you earn your living as an auditor for an insurance company. If your pleasure comes from windsurfing or hunting, you will want free distance vision more than if oil painting is your passion.

Think Ahead

Remember to think about presbyopia as you weigh these factors. Unless you can tolerate monovision, you must bear in mind that a successful two-eyed RK means glasses in your fifties, or sooner. You will not be able to read without glasses if both your eyes are 20/20: how much will that bother you? Unless you can be happy with one unoperated or undercorrected eye this is a consideration, except for high myopes who are usually looking forward to a -2 D or -3 D result— thus gaining, rather than losing, the ability to read easily without glasses.

Here's an angle some people think of: How much trouble do you expect in your future? If you are confident that society will remain stable and prosperous, and glasses or contacts will always be available, then you will not feel any need to avoid dependence on them on that score. But if you're a survivalist, you may want to take a day off from guerilla training to make sure you won't be stuck with no optician after the apocalypse.

Also, some people have a tendency to become involved in emergencies, like our friend whose boat sank on the way back from the hunting trip during which a bear knocked the stove over, set the tent on fire and chased him through the beehive and into the quicksand. Such folks may be anxious to have built-in focus correction.

It's How You See that Counts, Not How You Look. But...

Studies show that vanity is a very minor reason for RK, but perhaps it should be allowed a little influence. Darned if I can figure it out, though. As a homely dude with glasses, should I have been more or less anxious to be free of them than a Beautiful Person? On the one hand, the Beautiful Person might be the most eager to remove that last barrier to perfection, while a catfish is going to be ugly whether or not it wears spectacles. Then

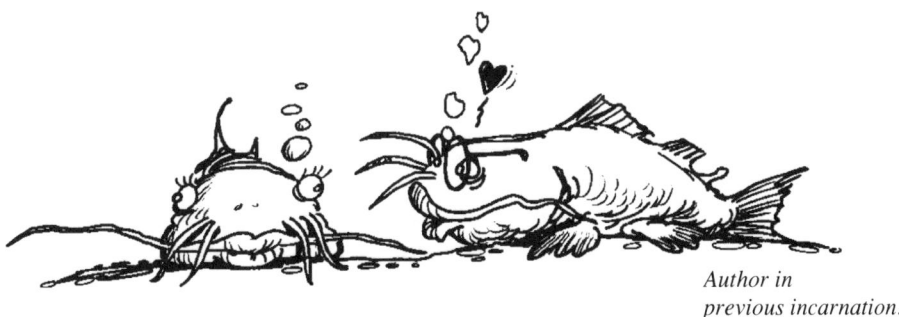

Author in previous incarnation.

again, try telling that to us catfish.

As you read case histories of RK and other refractive surgery, it does seem that the nearsighted person who feels trapped, unattractive, or hopelessly lonely may benefit from RK, especially if he or she considers the glasses to be a real handicap. The thrill of victory is certainly a boost under any circumstances. Obviously the operation won't change your life all by itself, but it could certainly be part of an honest effort to break out of a deep rut. Again, make sure that bad luck with RK won't devastate you.

Low-my: RK is OK for U and I

I'm a middling-low myope myself, so maybe I can be forgiven a few more paragraphs about the decision faced by my fellow lowies. We really do have a great new option in RK! If performed by an experienced surgeon, it is likely to be successful. If successful, it will eventually pay for itself many times over in savings on eyewear, particularly if the patient had an expensive love/hate relationship with contacts. The actual cutting involved will be much less than for severe myopia—possibly a quarter as much, considering the likelihood of only four incisions in one eye.

It's a happy fact that three fourths of all nearsighted people fall into the lower range. Most low myopes are very well-adjusted to nearsightedness; perhaps if it struck in adult years, like baldness, we'd be more outraged. But for those of us who dislike glasses and contacts, the opportunity to purchase such a good chance of improved vision for the price of a very used car is the bargain of a lifetime.

Yet even for the low myope, there is still a chance of not escaping glasses. There's a much smaller chance of coming out worse off than you started, and even a remote chance of serious loss of vision in one eye. And there is some inconvenience, discomfort, and expense to be borne. Certainly anyone who likes wearing glasses has no need for RK, and should ignore any enthusiastic bonehead who urges him to try it.

Cooling Your Jets

For most mildly or moderately nearsighted glasses-and-contact-haters the decision is not a matter of whether, but when—to go ahead now, or to wait. Here are some reasons for waiting:

You may want to make sure you've given contacts a fair trial.

It may take time to find a surgeon in your area who is proficient at the operation.

You may need some time to save up the money. See chapter 16.

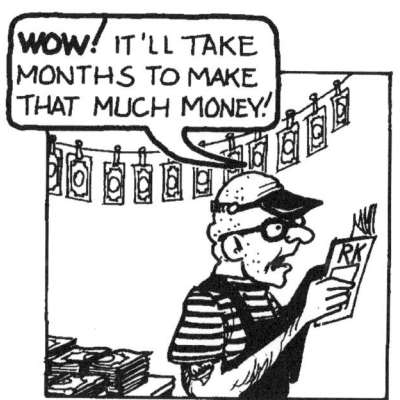

There may be no outstanding RK doc in your area, requiring extra money and time to visit one in another city.

The eighteen- or nineteen-year-old may be persuaded to wait another year or two, having refractions done annually, to make sure vision has completely stabilized.

The under-40 high myope also may want to wait a couple more years in hopes of getting a greater amount of correction. Now that's a patient patient.

Waiting for the New Model

Of course, the most common reason for holding off is probably the hope that the operation will become even more surefire, with less risk, cost, or inconvenience. This is a reasonable position, particulary for people in their early twenties. It is certainly possible that in ten or fifteen years, there could be substantial improvements.

The odds of hitting 20/20 could get much better. Over-correction might be prevented by pharmaceutical means or by the use of tiny sutures. The likelihood of losing vision in one eye might go from miniscule to unheard-of.

Maybe RK clinics like Professor Fyodorov's in Moscow will open here, with assembly-line setups—five surgeons in a row, each specializing in one portion of the operation. Maybe these clinics will charge less money. (Don't hold your breath.)

Even 'igher Eye-Tech, Mate

More enticing still, as we'll see in Chapter 19, is the possibility that laser cornea-sculpturing will pan out, and a computer-controlled excimer laser beam will shave a few microns off your central clear zone, to specifications. No incisions, no fl attened cornea, no big deal. Maybe this innovation will make RK obsolete.

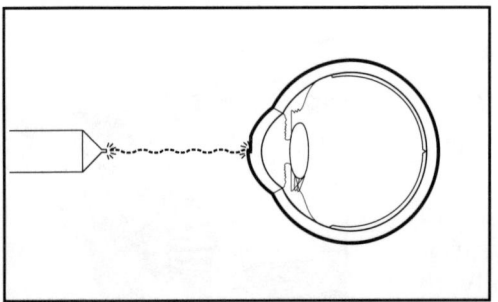

Cornea reshaping with an excimer laser

Then again, maybe not. Possibly this shaving of the crucial central zone will prove too hazardous. It will take many years to work out the bugs, and foolish actions by bureacrats and patent officials could snarl progress to a crawl. The F.D.A.'s authority over the new instrument promises no greased-lightning progress.

Certainly, anyone who doesn't mind waiting eight or ten years in hopes of an improved procedure should do so. Since there is absolutely no need to hurry, this decision can be made in the most leisurely manner—it is such a happy choice to ponder that it would be wasteful to hurry through it. You may want to do the further research suggested in chapter 17.

You Are Now Among the Best-Eyeducated People in the World

The next step for you low and moderate nearsighters, if you are seriously weighing RK, is to find your RK surgeon. Read Chapter 16! Then you need to present yourself for an examination and conversation, and only then can you make an informed decision.

I hope you enjoy the examination, and your discussions with your doctor—bring this book along, with markers to help you find areas where you have a question or concern. Take your time in making the decision; reread some of these last few chapters.

All you high myopes and astigmatic folks: onward to the next two chapters!

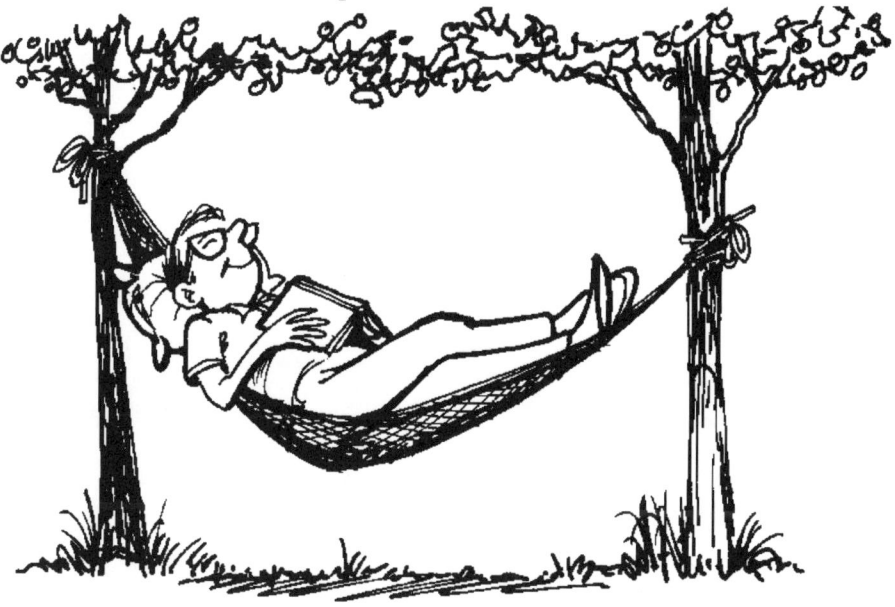

"Blind Without Glasses"?
High Myopia is Not Forever!

14

Well, me highly myopic hearties, it's just us now—the lowly-myopic types have left us. They don't know it, but to a great degree they owe the whole RK opportunity to the high myopes whose constant prodding, more than anything else, provoked the world's ophthalmologists to develop refractive surgery.

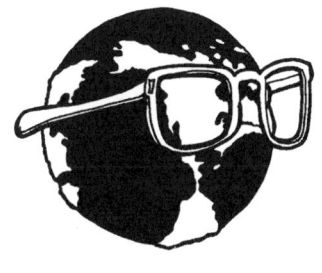

Something close to 2% of us are highly myopic. The old suspicion among optometrists that higher I.Q. and higher myopia often go together has recently been confirmed by a major study in Israel. Some professionals also believe that very-nearsighted people tend to be highly motivated, determined, perseverent. They make a strong lobby for advances in refractive ophthalmology.

We've seen that as the degree of myopia increases, the chances of complete success with RK go downhill. Older patients get significantly more nearsight-reduction, but for the under-forty high myope the odds of "success" drop off into pretty deep water.

Unless, of course, you consider a different definition of success. After all, the problem is not that the high myope is a lousy patient who responds badly to the operation, but that he often needs more cornea-flattening than the operation can provide. The -8 D person can obtain a five- or six-diopter correction just as easily as the -6 D person; it's just that the 8-diopter pilgrim would like to get a full 8 diopters of correction, and that's usually more than RK can deliver.

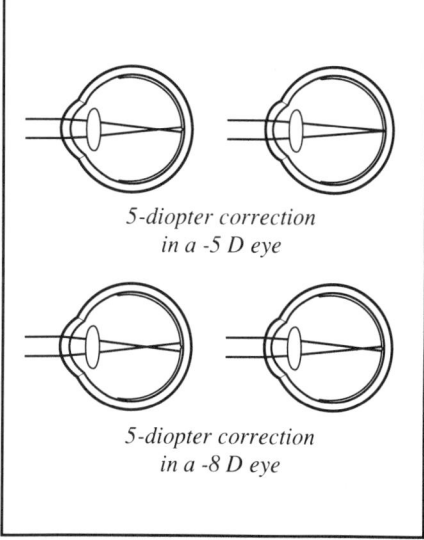

5-diopter correction in a -5 D eye

5-diopter correction in a -8 D eye

129

The Trend Toward Caution

A few years ago many surgeons would shoot for high amounts of correction, even in younger patients. They would use sixteen or even thirty-two incisions, small central clear zones, very deep incisions, or even intentionally perforate the inner cornea. But the results were often unsatisfactory: too much glare, irregular astigmatism, fluctuating vision, and large overcorrections occurred.

Nowadays, for a -8 D high myope in his or her thirties, for example, most surgeons will only aim for a six-diopter correction. They will only accept high-myopia patients who understand that they will still need the glasses of a mild myope, and are sure they'll be delighted with that outcome. A few may over-respond; if so they'll come away with 20/20, rather than be overcorrected.

Some of the RK specialists, who have done thousands of operations, have developed individualized techniques with which they often get very good results, and insist that they can shoot for high degrees of correction safely. But in the last few years the majority of RK surgeons have accepted that more than six diopters of flattening is not a realistic expectation except in older patients—the older the higher, with over ten diopters possible in the over-60 age group.

Mild Myopia: a Successful Result?

Surgeons say that many of their most delighted patients were high myopes who came away with low myopia. These are patients who go from absolute dependence on glasses to the sort of myopia that allows easy reading without glasses (for life), and is generally considered a minor nuisance by most people who have it.

It seems unfair: the low or moderate myope goes to RK with at least some hope of being freed from glasses, and will be at least a little disappointed if he isn't. Yet the high myope is hearing me say that even if he goes through the same hassle he should not hope to achieve 20/20 or even 20/40. Sure, it's unfair. Yet many professionals believe that the high myope who achieves low myopia has gained more than the low myope who achieves 20/40 or even 20/20. The reduction in visual distortion, the increase in image size, the normalization of appearance (because your eyes also appear more full-sized behind low-myopia glasses), and the escape from severe dependence are all greater in going from, say, -8D to -2D, than in going from low myopia to 20/20.

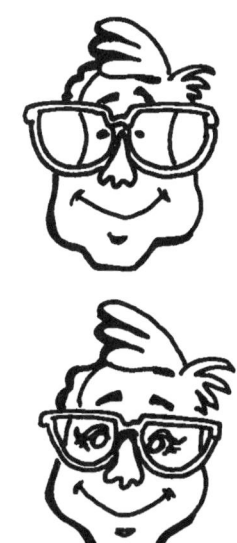

Sight for Survival

As a survival precaution, as well, the high-to-low successful RK makes more sense than a successful mild myopia-to-20/20 operation. And emergency-survival can be a crucial consideration for young American men and women—today's dangerous world presents a real possibility of someday needing to be able to drive a car, follow a trail, escape from violence, or exit a burning building without glasses.

While I was writing this chapter a very nearsighted 27-year-old woman was attempting to climb Mount Marcus Baker, a huge glacial peak near our city. She was inside a tent when she realized that the carbon monoxide fumes from her cookstove were making her dizzy—a situation in which death is just seconds away. Without her glasses, she tore out of the tent into a snowstorm "whiteout", and then was unable to find the tent again, and died of exposure within 35 feet of it. She was a very strong and experienced climber. So it's true that the combination of high myopia with dangerous circumstances can be deadly.

Some RK believers also cite a psychological benefit of high-myopia RK, even if the result is not perfect. Supposedly, the fact that the visual world is seen more full-sized, that one's appearance is more normal, and that the feeling of being dependent on a gadget is removed can have a heady effect on one's whole personality, and can lead to a sort of spiritual liberation. (Well, I believe it—after all, a mere cup of coffee can do the same for me.) Don't get me wrong—I'm certainly not trying to persuade anyone to have RK. My point is that for some highly myopic people, a less-than-20/40 result can still be a success, if that's the result they were expecting.

Making the Bullseye Wider

If the surgeon is attempting to correct high myopia to a perfect 20/20 or 20/40 result, the odds are not great: possibly a 15 % chance of 20/20, and a 30% or 40% chance of 20/40, with the odds increasing with the patient's age. (Young people, especially women, would have almost no chance of getting a full correction of more than 6 diopters, while a 50-year-old of either sex would have a much better chance.) If the goal is changed to "-2 D or better", the chances of that degree of success are much better.

For the six-to-ten-diopter high myope who is determined to escape high myopia, but doesn't demand complete correction, RK is presently the best bet. The laser-shaving technique which we'll discuss in Chapter 19 may offer a better way in eight or ten years, and if so, may work well as a fine-tuning technique for undercorrected RK patients. If I were highly myopic and hated it, I would consider a probably-undercorrected RK now, and keep monitoring the progress of new refractive techniques in hopes of a touch-up job at a future date. What I would not do is set my heart on complete escape from glasses, and badger my doctor for re-operation if I came away undercorrected.

Higher Yet: Myopia in the Teens and Twenties

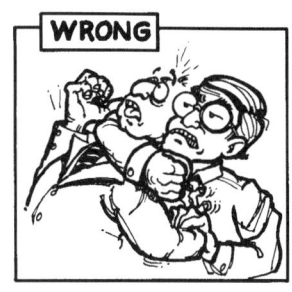

For "very high" myopia, above ten diopters (the most astronomical refractive surgery patient I've heard of had 49 surplus diopters) RK is not enough. Some older patients can get as much as thirteen diopters corrected with RK, but usually seven or eight is the limit without getting overly heroic.

Some people suffer from a progressive type of myopia, in which the eyeball continues to lengthen and myopia worsens steadily. Eventually, the retina may be stretched too far, and detaches or begins to degenerate, resulting in blindness. There is a surgical procedure to prevent this, called "scleral reinforcement".

This sort of "malignant" myopia is rare, but it's not uncommon for high myopia to be at least slightly progressive. It's a good idea to bring along your old eyewear prescriptions, or even the old glasses, when you visit a refractive-surgery ophthalmologist.

There are several alternative operations for very-high myopia currently in various stages of development.

Of course, RK could help. It will probably be able to correct six or seven diopters, depending on your age; if that's enough to be worthwhile, go for it. But for most very-high myopes, that much improvement is not sufficiently exciting. Naturally, they will be looking at the full-correction solutions, of which there are several.

The Non-RK Cornea-Flatteners

These operations work by flattening the cornea, like RK, but they involve removing, reshaping or installing thin slices of corneal tissue. They tend to be more difficult to perform, more unpredictable, and about twice as expensive as RK.

The "classic" high-myopia surgery, first developed almost 40 years ago by one of the honored founders of refractive surgery, Dr. Jose Barraquer of Colombia, is called Mypoic Keratomileusis. With this technique, a small disc of corneal tissue is planed off the surface of the cornea, frozen, lathed to a new, flatter shape, and then replaced on the cornea. Myopic keratomileusis is used mostly for errors in the -8 D to -15 D range.

The instruments required to do this are expensive, and exquisite skill is required, so only a few surgeons have adopted this procedure. The degree of predictability: perhaps a 70% chance of 20/40. It does have a long track record and there are several surgeons who are extremely experienced at it. Myopic Keratomileusis (MKM) is at this writing the most-used operation for very-high myopia; it is sometimes fine-tuned or enhanced by subsequent RK, which when performed after MKM has much more effect than usual. Of course, this is quite a bit of surgery on the little cornea.

Epi: the "Living Contact Lens"

A more recent solution is a related operation called myopic epikeratophakia (or "epi" for short.) A shallow circular incision is made in the outer cornea, and a little frisbee of donor-cornea tissue is set right on top of the patient's cornea, with the edges tucked into the circular incision. The patient's own cornea cells migrate into the donor

How to perform an MKM:

First, remove a disc of central cornea.

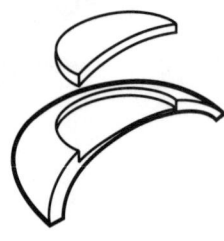

Then freeze the disc, and plane off part of the middle portion.

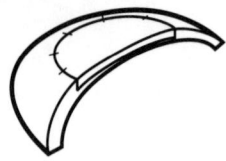

Then suture the disc back in place. Believe me, it's harder than it looks!

tissue, take up residence there among the stromal fibers, and make it part of you.

This procedure is reversible, at least in theory—the surgeon can remove the grafted disc if the result is unsatisfactory, and either admit defeat or try again. The patient's own cornea is still all there, and the optical zone is intact—usually.

"Epi" may become widely used eventually, but it will take a few more years to get all the bugs worked out—at present, the predictability is very poor and numerous problems have yet to be solved. For most highly myopic patients it would make sense to hold off another couple of years.

An Exciting New Approach

Dr. Luis Ruiz of the Barraquer Institute in Bogota has developed a new version of Keratomileusis called "Keratomileusis In Situ", which is being introduced in America by RK Pioneer Dr. Leo Bores of Scottsdale, Arizona. First, the surgeon planes off a disk of cornea tissue, less than half the thickness of the central cornea. This is set aside and a second, thinner disc is also planed off. The second disc is discarded, and the first is put back and sutured in place. The result is a much flatter cornea, resulting in up to 30 diopters of correction.

This appears to be a relatively safe operation, because it doesn't invade the interior of the eye and the tissue does not have to be frozen or lathed. Patients seem to recover rapidly, and in the first 48 patients, 59% achieved 20/40 vision or better. It will take awhile before this new procedure is thoroughly tested and proven, and awhile longer before very many American ophthalmologists have mastered it, but it looks good so far.

How to perform an 'Epi'

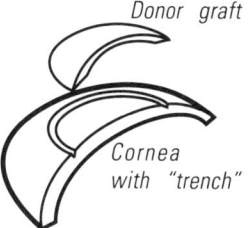
Donor graft
Cornea with "trench"

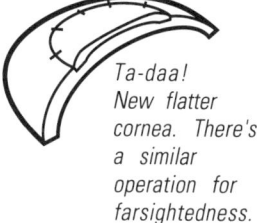
Ta-daa! New flatter cornea. There's a similar operation for farsightedness.

"But It's Not My Fault", Screamed the Lens

There is another, very different very-high-myopia operation called "clear-lens extraction". This is a cataract operation without a cataract: even though your lens is still perfectly clear, and quite innocent, it is removed—relieving you of its 15 unneeded diopters—and replaced with a much lower-powered artificial lens, or even a negative-powered one in extreme cases. This is a cut-and-dried procedure, a routine cataract operation—the anterior-segment surgeon's bread-and-butter.

So why isn't it done all the time to correct high myopia? Three main reasons:

Reason 1: With cataract surgery there is always about one chance in five hundred that the dreaded eye infection, endophthalmitis, will occur—and possibly destroy vision by damaging the retina. The reason for this high danger, much worse than with RK, is that cataract surgery invades the eye to remove the lens. With normal cataract removal, the alternative to surgery is certain blindness because of the clouded lens, so this risk is acceptable—but with clear lens extraction the alternative is merely continued nearsightedness.

Reason 2: There are several other problems that can develop, the most serious being retinal detachment, in which the retina begins to come unglued from the inside of the eyeball. It begins with a small hole or tear in the retina, which allows fluid to get behind the retina and start peeling it off the eyeball like wallpaper. If caught early this can often be cured, sometimes with a simple laser treatment. The high myope should have his eyes checked yearly, because the elongated eyeball that usually causes high myopia tends to increase the likelihood of retinal detachment. Major "invasive"

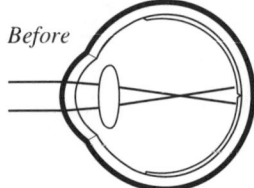

Before

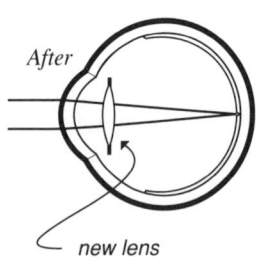

After

new lens

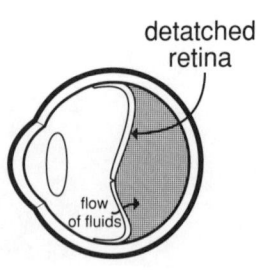

detached retina

flow of fluids

surgery such as lens extraction increases it further yet—in fact, there is something like a 7% chance of serious complications within five years of clear-lens extraction.

Instant Presbyopia

Reason 3: With the lens gone, accommodation is also lost forever. You will not be able to see far and also read with the same eye, without glasses. If you can handle monovision, of course, you can overcome this by having two different artificial lenses implanted: one for distance, and a stronger one in the other eye for reading. Still, this is not as nice as natural accommodation, because while one eye may be in focus on infinity and the other on twenty inches, that still leaves the middle distance poorly focused.

So the correction of high myopia by removing the natural lens and replacing it with a lower-powered artificial one offers excellent precision, but high risk and the loss of accommodation. For a sixty-year-old high myope with incipient cataracts, it may be an appealing prospect. For the younger patient who still enjoys accommodation, is not facing the risks of cataract surgery in any case, and has to consider the unknowns of the long term, clear-lens extraction is usually not too thrilling, although some extremely myopic patients have been very satisfied with it.

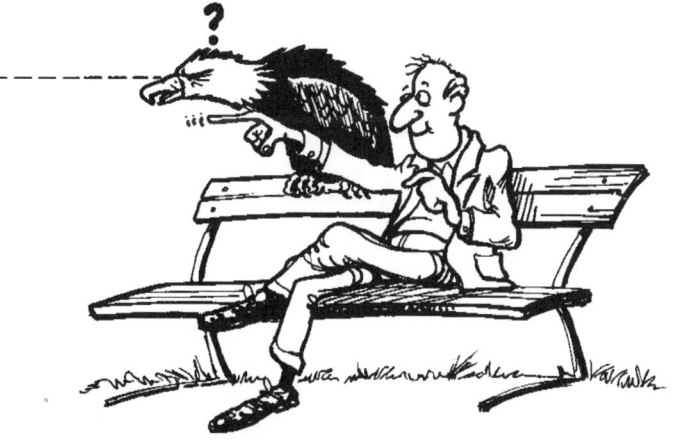

Born Too Soon?

Twenty years from now, possibly much sooner, there will probably be a completely satisfactory solution. If shaving of the central cornea with the excimer laser proves workable, then high myopia will be almost unheard-of in twenty years (or at least by the year 2020!) Please read Chapter 17 on future developments.

For now, the average higher myope is best advised to be patient, and not *a* patient, for a few more years. The clear-lens extraction is unappealing to younger people who hate to surrender their accommodation prematurely, and to any patient unwilling to take a risk of serious trouble. Keratomileusis and epikeratophakia are less risky and preserve accommodation, but they're less predictable. Of the two, Keratomileusis is more reliable and proven, but is also more expensive and not widely available. It's really only attractive to the few patients who are most anxious to escape from their myopia and can afford the cost, which runs from five thousand up. Quite possibly the in-situ keratomileusis will turn out to be the best of the non-invasive cornea-flattening techniques, but it's too soon to be sure.

So stay healthy, take care of your eyes, get regular check-ups, and save up some money! Follow the instructions in Chapter 17 on staying informed, and you will eventually be victorious.

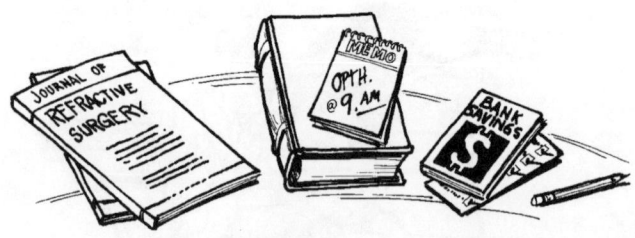

Another Ism We Could Do Without

15

Terrorism, extremism, astigmatism: who needs 'em? Once these 'isms get started they're mighty hard to get rid of, but it looks like refractive surgery will soon have astigmatism on the run.

People with astigmatism are known in the eye business as "astigmats", not astigmatists. People with low astigmatism often don't even know they have it—how many people ever read their eyeglass prescriptions?—but highly astigmatic people certainly know it and hate it. They are the bane and sorrow of eye professionals, because their problems are so varied and baffling.

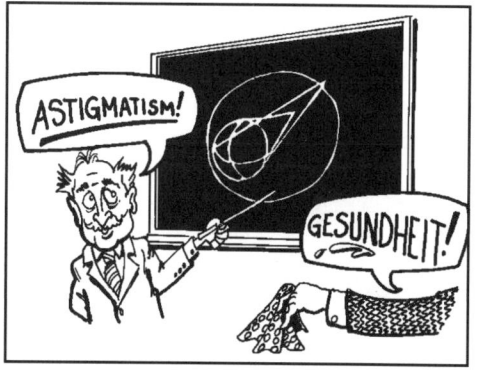

Joke no. 724, Volume XXVI

Astigmatism is a weird Greek word meaning "without a point", for the astigmatic eye does not focus upon a single point on the retina. Although some astigmatism is occasionally caused by the lens, usually the cornea is to blame—the problem being that its face is not quite radially symmetrical: instead of being round like a bowl, it's slightly ovoid, like the side of a football or the back of a teaspoon. (Were it not for spoons and footballs, astigmatism would be impossible to describe.)

The "long meridian" of the cornea is less steeply curved, and therefore has less refractive power than the short, or steeper, meridian. Even though the ovalness is microscopic, the resulting image cast on the retina is also oval, instead of a point as in the 20/20 eye, or a round disk as in myopia and hyperopia.

A Football Lies On Its Side, As a Rule

Usually, the steeper meridian of the cornea is more or less vertical, and the flatter meridian is horizontal. This is called "with-the-rule" astigmatism. When the steep meridian is horizontal and the flatter meridian is vertical, that's called "against-the-rule" astigmatism. With-the-rule is better to have: easier to fit with contacts and more bearable in general. There is also "oblique" astigmatism, in which the two meridians form a diagonal X instead of a cross.

With all of these, the steeper axis is at right angles to the flatter axis. When the two meridians don't form a 90-degree angle, which is fortunately rare, you have "irregular" astigmatism. This can be a troublesome problem, impossible to completely correct with glasses.

Curiously, as the years go by the eye sometimes flattens in the vertical axis—that is, mild with-the-rule astigmatism can go away on its own, and non-astigmatic eyes sometimes become against-the rule astigmatic in later life.

The traditional solution to astigmatism is glasses, with lenses that are slightly cylindrical, instead of spherical—that is, they add or subtract more power in one meridian than another, to "even out" the eye's focusing. For with-the-rule astigmatism, the "cylinder" runs horizontally, so it subtracts power from the too-strong vertical axis but has no effect on the horizontal axis.

Often, astigmatism accompanies myopia, and the cylindrical component is combined with the concave component when the lenses are ground. Sometimes astigmatism accompanies hyperopia (farsightedness) or stands alone, with no other error.

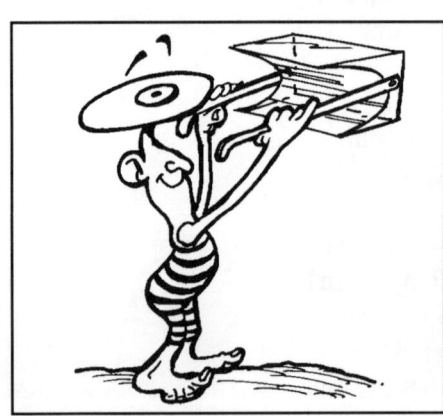

With-the-rule Astigmatism meets its match: horizontal-axis cylindrical lens

I'd rather eat a bee than have to go over astigmatism prescriptions again, but my editor says I don't have the option. Maddeningly, the profession uses two different ways of describing astigmatism, called plus form and minus form.

Here's the minus-form prescription for a person with three diopters of myopia and two diopters of with-the-rule astigmatism: -3.00 - 2.00 x 180 degrees. So this eye is really three diopters myopic horizontally, but five diopters nearsighted in the steeper, vertical meridian.

Here's the plus-form description of the same eye: -5.00 + 2.00 x 90 degrees. Says the same thing: 5 diopters myopic at the vertical axis, but only 3 diopters (-5 + 2) at the horizontal axis.

You can tell whether you're looking at plus form or minus form by looking at the sign in front of the second number (the 2 in this example). A minus sign means minus form. In this book when we say, for example, "three diopters of myopia and two diopters of astigmatism", we're thinking minus form: -3.00 - 2.00 x 180.

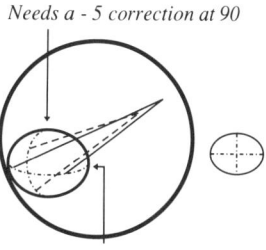

Needs a - 5 correction at 90

Needs a - 3 correction at 180

A Terror of an Error

If uncorrected, astigmatism can be very annoying. It makes you accommodate excessively, which exhausts the ciliary muscle, and causes blurred vision, squinting, tired eyes after close work, head-tilting, and frontal headaches. Even low degrees of astigmatism may cause transient blurriness during reading or other close work, which is relieved by closing or rubbing the eyes.

High degrees of astigmatism, especially against-the-rule and oblique astigmatism, can be devilishly hard to correct well with glasses, and often the patient has to put up with considerable distortion and less than 20/20 vision. Such astigmats are acknowledged by all ophthalmologists to be truly handicapped by their visual errors.

A Mob of Astigmats with Torches is after Baron von Contact

Contact lenses are harder to fit for more-than-mildly astigmatic patients than for simple myopes or hyperopes. Generally, normal soft contacts don't work, because they conform to the shape of the astigmatic cornea. Hard contacts and gas-permeable contacts sometimes will do the trick, if the patient can tolerate the "astigmatic rock"—the tendency of the hard lens to wobble on the astigmatic cornea like a table with a short leg. There are also "toric" soft contacts, which are specially shaped to fit the astigmatic eye and work well for some people. The astigmatic contact-seeker needs a particularly talented ophthalmologist and/or optometrist, and may have to go through several to find one with the patience and know-how required. It's worth the trouble—much as we like to kid the poor Baron, contact lenses are a godsend for many astigmatic people and often give them much better vision than glasses can provide.

Refractive Surgery Tackles the Football-Shaped Cornea

Severe astigmatism has often been a side-effect of cataract surgery—after the cornea is lifted up like a flap to remove the cloudy lens and stitched in place again, it sometimes heals unevenly and becomes too steep in one meridian. So eye surgeons have been trying to correct astigmatism with incisions on the cornea for over 100 years. Thanks to RK and the coming-of-age of corneal microsurgery, they are now getting pretty good at it.

Basically, surgery for astigmatism attempts to flatten the steep meridian of the cornea, to make it as flat as the flatter meridian. To do this, special "relaxing incisions" are placed across the steep meridian. These incisions can also cause slight steepening of the flatter meridian, a phenomenon called "coupling". The sum of the two effects equals the total effect in decreasing the astigmatism.

As with RK for myopia, it is possible to have an overcorrection. However, for the astigmatic patient, this results not in farsightedness, but in residual astigmatism in the opposite meridian—for example, three diopters of against-the-rule astigmatism might be overcorrected, and leave the patient with one diopter of with-the-rule astigmatism, a big improvement. In this sense, astigmatic keratotomy is considered more forgiving than RK. Since against-the-rule astigmatism is a greater nuisance, surgeons lean toward overcorrecting when they operate on it, whereas for with-the-rule they lean toward undercorrection.

Generally, astigmatism without myopia or with low myopia is more bothersome than with high myopia, and it's also easier to correct with surgery. The surgeon takes all these factors into account when he plans your surgery. Obviously, if you're astigmatic you need a doc who's experienced in this tricky area of refractive surgery.

Rally 'Round the Flag Incisions

Mild astigmatism associated with myopia can usually be corrected quite easily as part of the RK procedure. In fact, for some reason the RK'd cornea sometimes tends to flatten more vertically than it does horizontally, and so corrects small degrees of with-the-rule astigmatism—or even induces a small amount of against-the-rule astigmatism. Also, with-the-rule astigmatism usually diminishes with age. So in younger patients it is probably best not to try to correct mild with-the-rule astigmatism, up to a diopter or so.

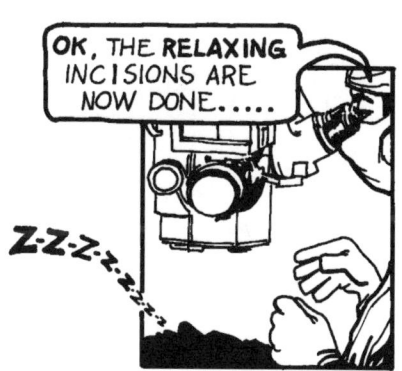

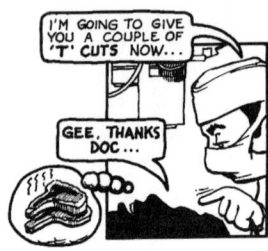

When mild astigmatism does need to be corrected, small "flag" incisions or transverse incisions—the docs call them "T-cuts"—are added to the RK procedure. The precise technique used varies from surgeon to surgeon, much more than with the basic RK—some use small, close-to-the-center flag incisions added to the RK incisions, while others may use longer, more peripheral incisions, sometimes installed after the RK cuts have healed. Most surgeons get reasonably good results, and most patients are pleased—having been warned in advance that they will probably not be relieved of all their astigmatism.

Highly astigmatic patients should also be warned that in the post-op period they will experience considerably more pain, light-sensitivity and glare than with a simple RK. As the degree of astigmatism increases, so do the number and size of the transverse or flag incisions—while only two may be needed to correct three diopters, as many as four are required for higher degrees. More incisions mean more discomfort afterwards, and more glare and light-sensitivity in the recovery period.

Overly Oval Eyes are a Challenge

For severe astigmatism, above 3.5 diopters, and astigmatism without myopia, the picture is less promising. The simple T-cuts are not sufficiently effective, and the challenge is to find a set of incisions that will yield an effect great enough to do the job, without harming the cornea or causing complications.

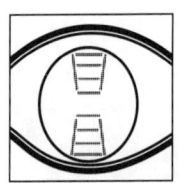

"Modified Ruiz Procedure" incision pattern

Several operative strategies are being used. The most popular at this point is the modified Ruiz procedure, which combines radial RK-type cuts with transverse incisions.

Originally, the innermost rung of the stepladder was connected to the radial incision on either side, but this caused healing problems, so now the rule is that no incisions may cross one another. For pure astigmatism, the Ruiz procedure is used alone; when myopia is also present, RK is combined with a Ruiz procedure (sometimes with a waiting period in between). A number of surgeons are getting very good at the Ruiz procedure. Usually the surgeon will use a special device which allows him to monitor the roundness of the cornea changing as the operation proceeds.

This operation does reduce astigmatism dramatically most of the time, but the result is less predictable than with RK for myopia—within 1 diopter of the desired result perhaps 70% of the time. Also, generally speaking, this severe-astigmatism surgery causes more discomfort, light-sensitivity and glare than does RK-plus-flag-incision surgery, and it may take longer for vision to stabilize afterwards.

You Aren't Getting Older, You're Getting Better Correction

As with RK, more correction is possible in older patients. At twenty or thirty, it's hard for the patient to get more than a six-diopter correction, while at sixty it may be possible to obtain nine or ten diopters of effect. Also, the older patient probably has a more stabilized error, not likely to change much with passing years.

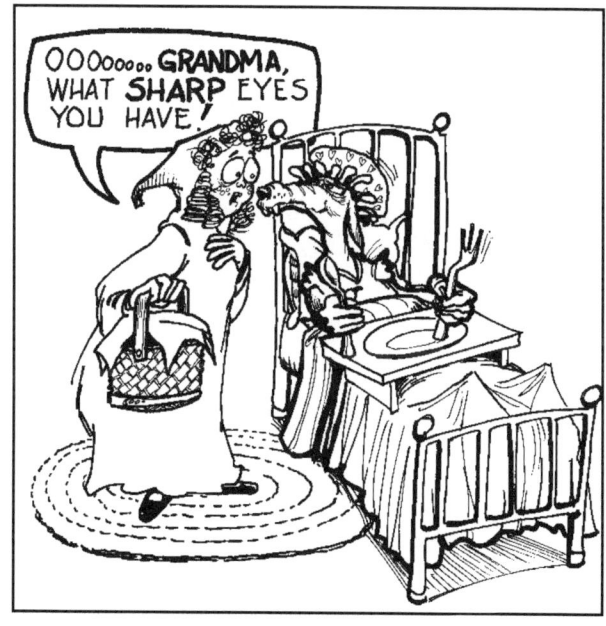

The nerves in the cornea enter radially from the periphery, so the transverse incisions used for astigmatism tend to sever more of them than the radial RK incisions. Astigmatic Keratotomy (AK) patients therefore often lose some sensitivity for several months after surgery, which may have some effect on tear-film production and healing, so these patients should be particularly alert to any inflammation or other problem which may develop.

Astigmatism surgery is probably less predictable than RK, and is more in need of further research and analysis. Most highly astigmatic people who can get 20/20 vision with glasses or contact lenses will probably stick with them for a few more years, and only those who cannot be satisfactorily corrected with glasses or contact lenses will seek the surgical alternative.

Such people should make sure to find a surgeon with ample experience in astigmatism correction. Read Chapter 17 and do some further research. Corneal optics is very interesting science, combining math, physics and two or three other disciplines.

Grounds for Ophtimism

Fortunately, several outstanding surgeons are pouring a lot of time and energy into astigmatism-correction research. You have to admire the determination and intelligence of these researchers, whose efforts are resulting in more reliable and standardized means of defeating astigmatism. They are advancing the science at an astonishing rate.

Next, we'll talk a bit about finding a good surgeon and (shudder) paying him.

Finding the Doc and the Dollars   16

About a tenth of American ophthalmologists perform RK, and more are learning it—"adding it to their armamentarium" is the medical phrase—every year. Still, this is a surprisingly small number, and you probably wonder why so few are able to offer such a valuable service to their patients. There are several reasons, of which perhaps the most important is financial: few hospitals are equipped for RK, and it costs too much for most surgeons to set up an operating room of their own. Another good reason: RK is an extremely demanding operation, much more skill-intensive than, say, cataract surgery.

The RK Controversy

Of course, RK is still controversial. After all, it's an operation performed on a healthy eye, an eye which usually can already deliver good vision with the aid of glasses. This offends many ophthalmologists who have spent countless hours convincing patients that there is nothing wrong with wearing glasses, that nearsightedness is not a flaw or handicap. These doctors may not appreciate how much some of us hate being nearsighted.

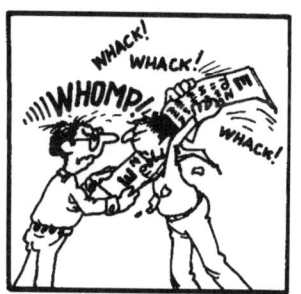

Many doctors also opposed contacts for years, and this may have been justifiable considering the drawbacks of the old hard lenses. Eventually nearly all eye professionals accepted contacts as a slightly more hazardous solution to nearsightedness, appropriate for patients who disliked glasses. It will be some years before RK is accepted in the same spirit, as something some patients want.

There are also some less respectable reasons for opposing RK. Most powerful is the age-old

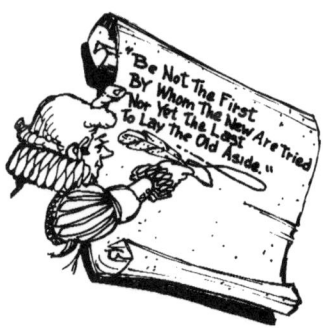

Many surgeons believe old Alexander Pope said it best

fear and hatred of new innovations, the same deep-seated loathing that caused 19th-Century surgeons to attack Semmelweiss and Lister for suggesting that surgeons caused infections by operating with dirty hands. In the Seventies, this closed-minded attitude caused a civil war that split the profession between those who felt that cataract patients should be content with thick glasses, and those who favored implanting artificial lenses as part of the operation. The old-fashioned surgeons opposed that wonderful innovation ferociously, going so far as to seek national legislation against it. They lost, and today nearly all cataract patients get implants, and are freed from "cataract glasses".

Who Wants to Go Back to School?

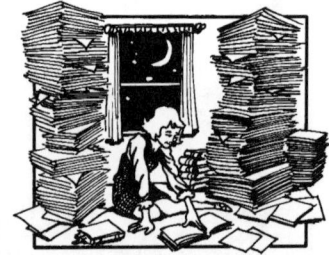

Before he can perform RK, a surgeon must spend weeks learning the procedure and practicing on animal and cadaver eyes. He may have to travel far from his home to study under an expert. There is also an enormous amount of reading to be done. A lot has been written about RK, and the surgeon has to read most of it. Many doctors who disparage RK have not kept up with the literature and have no idea of the recent progress.

It is true that many ophthalmologists have comfortable working arrangements with optometrists and opticians, and it has been speculated that these setups make some doctors oppose any alternative to glasses. I don't think this is a significant factor.

Since most myopes are content with glasses, and RK is never an emergency need, it is not necessary for most eye surgeons to offer it. No one should criticize those who don't. The ophthalmologists who flatly condemn the operation and won't admit that it's right for anybody, however, are doing their patients a disservice. If your ophthalmologist takes such an attitude, and won't even refer you to an RK-capable surgeon, I'd consider finding a new ophthalmologist. This doctor's tightly closed mind may not serve you well in other eye matters, either.

You Can Find One

Fortunately, there are quite a few ophthalmologists who do perform RK. Is there such a one in your area? Probably, especially if you live near a large metropolis. Almost certainly, if you live in the Sunbelt, where RK is generally more common than in the Northeast. How do you find one?

It takes some effort. One angle is to call the nearest major teaching hospital—usually affiliated with a university—and ask to speak with the chief resident in ophthalmology. Explain that you are seeking one of the top RK surgeons in your area, and with any luck he'll suggest someone, or tell you who else could advise you.

If you already have an ophthalmologist, but he or she does not perform RK, this doctor may be able to suggest a top RK tiger. Checking the names of authors of articles or chapters in the books listed in Chapter 17 may help you find a surgeon with expertise in the particular problem you have—high myopia, severe astigmatism, farsightedness etc. Your ophthalmologist will often have these books and periodicals. A few hours of research can work wonders.

Some patients seek out a famous surgeon who has published lots of papers or done thousands of operations. Some of these are indeed among the finest surgeons.

Of course, many ophthalmologists who have not done hundreds of operations, or built great reputations by their writing or research, are extremely talented and do superb work. Also, it is true that some of the thousand-operation RK specialists have accumulated their huge experience by "pushing" the operation, instead of taking a neutral and objective stance, or by accepting candidates most surgeons would discourage.

Top Anterior-Segment Surgeons Only Need Apply

My own surgeon, Dr. Marvin Grendahl of Anchorage, Alaska, had performed fewer than fifty RK's when mine was done. However, when I made inquiries I found that he was one of the most experienced and respected eye surgeons in the state, with a long and impressive surgical record. I was extremely impressed by his calm, professional manner, his patience, and the unsalesmanlike way in which he presented the alternatives. He didn't promise the moon. He strongly urged that I not have both eyes done—it was he who introduced me to monovision. And the efficiency and competence of his staff impressed me. I decided that Dr. Grendahl was the kind of surgeon who would probably perform the operation in a conservative, painstaking, and meticulous way.

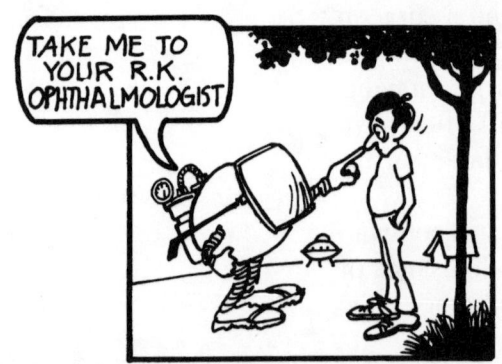

If you have a hunch that your local eye doc is an unusually talented surgeon and can give you an excellent RK, you should do a little research. In every city there are a relatively small number of ophthalmologists who do most of the "anterior segment" surgery, which includes all the things that go wrong with the cornea, iris, and lens. All anterior segment surgery is fairly tricky work. Its bread-and-butter is the removal of cataracts, the clouded lenses that eventually bedevil most senior citizens, accompanied by installation of the above-mentioned artificial intra-ocular lenses. A surgeon who has a reputation as a top hand at anterior segment surgery is more likely to be good at RK than one whose reputation is only average or who specializes in another area, or is more of a generalist.

You want the kind of surgeon to whom non-surgical ophthalmologists refer their surgical patients, and that's one way to confirm your tiger. Call a couple of ophthalmologists and ask them if Dr. X has a reputation as a top anterior-segment surgeon. Just like that—with a promise of confidentiality. If the answer is not a firm yes, look elsewhere.

On the average, a doctor's first dozen or so RK patients have worse odds of getting satisfactory results. Surgeons use the phrase "learning curve" to describe the improving results that are obtained as experience is accumulated, and there is probably no operation in which experience is so important as RK. With most operations, millimeters count—with RK, microns count. (Microns are thousandths of a millimeter.)

If the Doc gets Annoyed, Get Another Doc

You can also inquire as to the specifics of your surgeon's training in RK. Also, ask if you can see a complete list of your doctor's RK patients, and pick five names at random to call for references. This may violate your surgeon's regard for his patients' privacy; if so, offer to let his office call the ones you picked first to make sure they don't mind. Make sure to find out how many operations your doctor has done, over how long a span—the longer the better—and if yours is a special problem, what his experience is with that problem. Don't be embarrassed about being so nosy—after all, you are placing your most precious possession in his care.

You Can't Study for the Exam, but You Can Study the Examiner

Often you will get some clues during the pre-RK exam. Was it exhaustively thorough and complete? Did the doctor try to push you toward RK? (If so, back off.) Was he honest about RK's limitations, and willing to help you prepare for imperfect results by simulating them with lenses? Was he willing to help you test for monovision tolerance? Was he eager to answer questions, and able to relate to you as a person, not just a pair of nearsighted eyes? Ideally, the examination should be so thorough as to leave you slightly exhausted, and the doc should let you ask questions until he is in a similar state.

The literature you receive from the doctor may also give some clues, especially if he's prepared it himself. It should be thorough, especially with regards to the limitations and unpredictability of RK, and not too boosterish. This book, which stresses the limitations and promotes a conservative, painstaking approach, is considered too objective by some surgeons—immodest as it sounds, I would say that if the doc loaned or gave you this copy, that speaks very well of his objectivity and his willingness to have his patients know both sides of the picture.

You Operate on Both Eyes at Once, and Guarantee 20/20?
Thanks, but No Thanks, Dr. Rambo

Some surgeons actively promote RK, and even advertise it, and that seems fair since most nearsighted people are still unaware of this new option. However, it's important that this investment not compromise the surgeon's objectivity. A good surgeon should never "sell" RK to the individual patient—the doctor's persuasive skill should be concentrated on convincing you of the importance of following instructions before and after RK, convincing you that you may not get 20/20 or even 20/40, and that you may be overcorrected, have fluctuating vision, or conceivably experience a more serious complication.

The doctor should "sell" you those facts and make sure you have truly "bought" them. There is a fine line between telling you all about this exciting new option and pushing you toward it, and if he crosses that line repeatedly you should cease to trust his objectivity and judgement. The ophthalmologist should also support your interest in monovision, to the extent even of helping you get a half-strength contact lens for testing, if you desire.

Make sure that the surgeon you choose, be he a famous Grey Eminence or your tennis buddy, agrees with your idea of the ideal RK—which, if you agree with me, means a cautious approach: one eye only, if possible, or the non-dominant eye slightly undercorrected. Maximum wait between the two eyes—**never** both the same day. A slightly undercorrecting operative plan, in hopes that if it doesn't hit the bullseye it will come up short—an undercorrection, possibly fixable by re-operation—and not overshoot, resulting in hard-to-fix and even-harder-to-get-used-to farsightedness. It's a conservative approach, more trouble for the patient, and less profitable to the ophthalmologist, meaning you may have to pay a little more than for a "go for the gusto" approach—but it's worth it.

Which brings us to another interesting subject—paying for it.

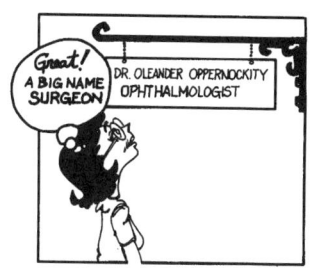

Warning: There are some surgeons out there who may put their own profit ahead of their patients' well-being. Remember that neither the FDA nor anyone else regulates eye surgery, so you must be careful!

Money Matters with RK

One thing that is not a consideration in choosing a surgeon is price. You don't take bids on RK! It's a relatively cheap surgery in any case, and the difference of a few hundred dollars should not be a factor.

The price for RK surgery averages about $1500 per eye. The lowest I've heard of is $800; the highest, $1800. It might make sense for the surgeon to charge more for the first eye, since half the battle is examining and educating the patient, but few surgeons have such a policy. The monovision patient is getting off easy, it seems.

Patients who expect to have both eyes operated on will want to make sure the financing is well squared away for both, prior to the first operation. You don't want to get stuck for a year or two with badly mismatched eyes. If you are paying the bill yourself, and a period of tight money is threatening, pay for both at the start. On the positive side, RK is one thing nobody can seize, repossess or sell at auction! On the downside, your pawnbroker won't be interested either.

As we have seen, many surgeons prefer to be cautious with their planning, and accept a high probability of undercorrection followed by touch-up surgery, in hopes of avoiding irreparable overcorrection. That's a fine approach, but who pays for the extra surgery, if required? You'll want to find out your surgeon's policy—some charge nothing extra; if so they must raise the basic price to cover this added cost. Others charge an operating-room fee, or some fraction of the cost of the original operation. All of these are fair deals. Generally, the doctors who operate in hospitals have less flexibility in charging for re-operations.

Insurance and RK

Will your insurance cover RK? Only your surety knows for sure, of course. Strangely, RK is more likely to be covered in the Southwest than in the rest of the country. Other important factors:

Type of policy—some carriers cover RK in an individual policy, but not in a group policy.

Specific exclusion—some carriers normally cover RK unless specifically excluded in your employer's policy.

Medical necessity—some carriers won't pay unless the surgery is deemed medically necessary for you, a case-by-case determination. This would depend on your degree of trouble with glasses and contact lenses. Generally, it is recognized that higher degrees of myopia, and even moderate degrees of astigmatism, are not fully correctable with glasses, so anyone with these problems who is unable to tolerate contacts should certainly be covered for RK as a medical necessity. Many people suffer from frontal headaches, sinus troubles, TMJ syndrome (jaw pain) and other conditions which make glasses extremely uncomfortable; these would make RK a medical necessity.

Many ophthalmologists feel that such special considerations are not essential—that nearsightedness and astigmatism are eye abnormalities warranting medical correction to meet the patient's needs, the same as any unwanted abnormality of any other part of the body. A club-footed man is not expected to forego surgery because crutches are available. You may find your ophthalmologist to be a strong ally in this battle, if it arises—he or she can write a letter to your carrier explaining your need for the surgery, for starters.

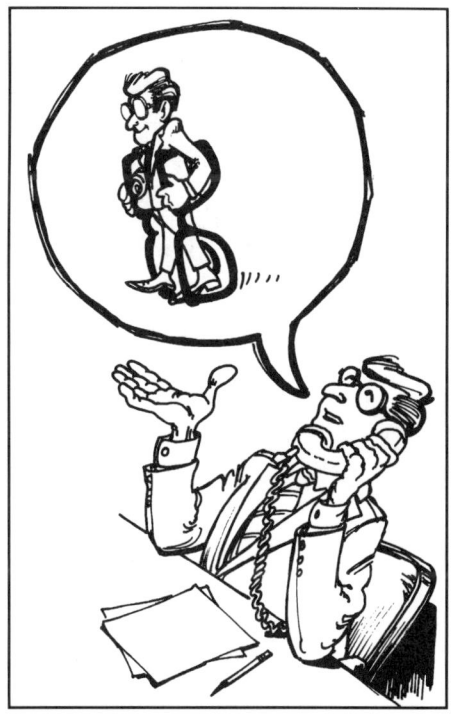

The procedures for high myopia, astigmatism and farsightedness are more likely to be covered than RK, because these errors are less common and more devilish than low myopia. These operations tend to cost more, too—roughly twice as much as RK.

Rock of Gibraltar, Cleft for Me

You should contact your carrier to determine its policy toward RK. Don't take anything for granted when dealing with insurance companies! Get it in writing, either way, and if they say no, insist that they tell you in writing exactly where in the policy RK is excluded. They may have a change of heart. Many RK patients have taken carriers to small claims court, and won. By the way, the surgical code number for RK is 6576052.

RK and the Army, Part II

Retired Army personnel and dependents of Army personnel can have RK performed for free at Fitzsimmons Army Medical Center in Aurora, Colorado, near Denver. Dr. Cornell, the surgeon in charge of this program, reports that the roughly 100 patients treated so far have been very happy, and so has the Army. This is a research program, so each patient must agree to the protocol, including checkups. Patients have come from all over the United States. The Navy and the Air Force may soon set up similar programs, so if you might be eligible, check with them to see if Uncle Sam will help you Be All that You Can Be, visually speaking.

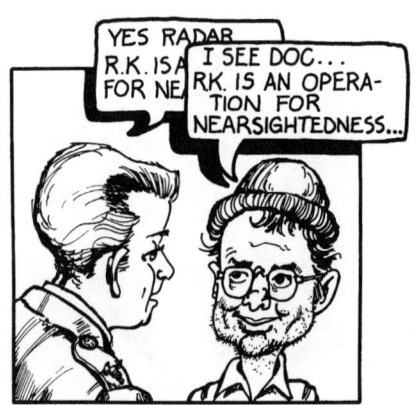

It makes sense for Uncle Sam, too—after all, the only other country that uses RK as much as America is the Soviet Union. And as our nation's largest employer, the army has more to gain from RK than any other institution. Who knows—maybe someday RK will be offered as an inducement to enlist.

Moscow This Ain't: We Pay Our Way in the USA

Alas! For many of us there is no one to pay for RK but ourselves. It was that way for me, and although it cost only a third as much as the bridge my dentist installed the year before, it was still a lot of money.

A good way to pay for RK is to set up a "Christmas fund" type of savings account and pay into it what you can afford. Twenty-five bucks a week will do the trick in a year or two, depending on whether you need both eyes corrected. This gives you time to choose the best surgeon, test for monovision tolerance, and do further research if you like (see next chapter).

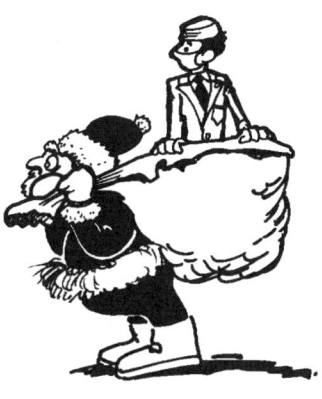

After all, you've put up with myopia for this long—another year won't kill you. Just take it one step at a time, patiently: choose a surgeon, have the pre-RK exam, get a second opinion if you like, and make up your mind. If it's thumbs-up, set up a special account and be religious about it, and you're on your way.

Next, let's take a look at what the future holds for RK and refractive surgery.

We'll All Have 20/20 by 2020
The Future and How to be Part of It   17

In 1985, I decided that Radial Keratotomy had been refined enough to suit me. Considering the mildness of my myopia and the severity of my dislike for glasses and contacts, I was satisfied with the state of the RK art as it stood then.

As we've seen, however, RK is still not perfect enough to suit all nearsighted people, and many prefer to watch and wait a little longer. This is even more likely to be the case for those who seek the new surgical procedures for high myopia, astigmatism, and farsightedness, which are evolving even faster. What you have learned from 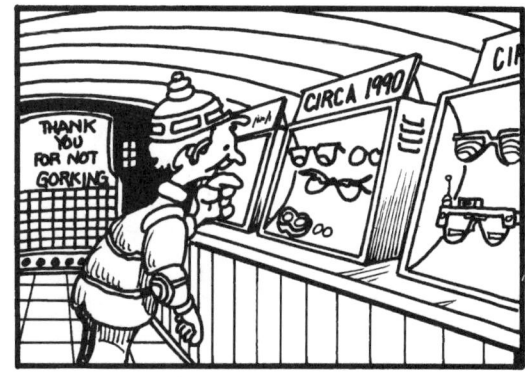 this book will enable you to understand the breakthroughs as they happen, and come to a sensible compromise between waiting for the perfect solution and enjoying as many years of improved vision as possible.

Nearly everyone in the field agrees that someday, all the common refractive errors will be routinely corrected by microsurgery. Unfortunately, that's about where agreement ends. Most authorities won't even guess when this happy day will dawn, except for a few who smile and say "2020."

It's not even possible to say for sure how long RK will continue to the best method for correcting mild and moderate nearsightedness, as it unquestionably is today. That depends on how much RK can be improved, and on how well the alternatives pan out—especially the laser possibilities that are just beginning to be explored.

All We Ask is Perfection

We've looked at RK honestly, without benefit of rose-colored glasses, and faced the fact that although it is usually successful, it's far from surefire. Even for low-myopia patients there is a significant chance of not achieving good vision. The possibility of overcorrection, the smaller chance of fluctuating vision, and the even more remote danger of a serious complication must be recognized. There's no doubt that RK will continue to be improved, and possibly some major improvements could come within the next five or ten years.

Perhaps four fifths of nearsighted people are in the RK range, but members of the highly-myopic minority are often the ones who want correction the most. So RK's main shortcoming is probably the fact that it can only provide five to six diopters of "anti-myopia", or more if you're older.

Possible means of increasing the operation's flattening power include drugs to slow the healing process or promote collagen growth in the incisions. Several new drugs made available by recombinant DNA technology are being investigated. There is also the idea of "corneal mortar", a substance that could be packed into the incisions, preventing regression while they heal.

But Shall We Overcome Overcorrection?

For us low and moderate myopes and for older folks with somewhat higher myopia, RK is powerful enough, so the main problem is the lack of predictability—the chance of not getting satisfactory uncorrected vision. A partial solution to this problem has evolved: the cautious, rather-have-to-operate-twice-than-get-overcorrected approach. But some patients continue to come away still nearsighted, or overcorrected into farsightedness. New methods of improving the accuracy of the correction are needed, and are being pursued.

Continued improvement in the tools and technology is sure to help. For instance, a new method of locating the visual axis has recently been published that may make the method we described obsolete. More accurate knives are being developed—that could be a big help, since variations in depth of incision are a major cause of unpredictable results. Better methods of visualizing the cornea's shape and curvature, including the curvature of its inner face, are also being developed.

If Only We All Were Exactly Alike

Better understanding of the variations between individual corneas should lead to greater predictability. The foundation of science is the belief that everything is caused, that nothing "just happens". The factors that cause some people's eyes to over-respond or under-respond to RK should be discoverable beforehand, and "factored in" to adjust the effect of the operation.

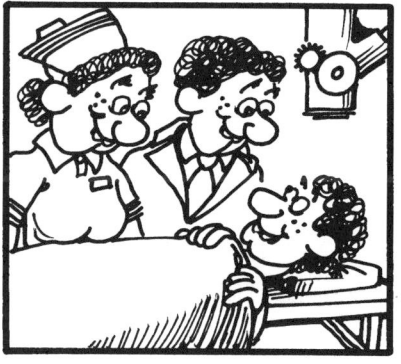

Even if your cornea's size and shape could be measured precisely, a great unknown remains: your cornea's own particular nature, it's cellular individuality. Like all of any person's body, your cornea is a unique and inscrutable community of little citizens, toiling away at tasks we can barely guess at, and officiously regulating such things as healing and rigidity. There is an intricate system of flow and feedback at work, chemicals being channeled, molecules throwing switches and getting blocked or admitted, all in accordance with the built-in instructions compiled in our DNA by the uncounted generations of survivors behind us. A field of biology called "channel theory" may lead the way to a better understanding of how this molecular activity works, and then the docs will be able to measure variations between individuals.

In Search of Fine-Tuning

RK's effectiveness results, at least in part, from the fact that the incisions don't close tight after the knife has passed, but "gape" slightly—and the wider they gape while they heal, the more the peripheral cornea bulges and the inner cornea flattens. So it seems likely that overcorrected RK's could be "brought back" toward perfection by tightening the incisions together, by means of tiny sutures (stitches). Dr. Richard L. Lindstrom of the University of Minnesota Medical School is currently investigating this approach. If it works well, this could be the answer to RK's single most common complication.

The use of drugs to enhance or diminish the effect of the operation is sometimes tried, but not always effective, and the use of steroids for long periods has caused cataracts in at least a couple of cases. With a little luck, new medicinal means may be found to adjust the post-RK focus.

There are now hundreds of surgeons performing RK, and many of them are trying hard to improve it in dozens of large and small ways. In ten years it will certainly be improved over its current state of art. But will the improvements be worth ten years of putting up with one's pre-RK myopia? Beats me.

Will The Laser Take Over?

RK may eventually be replaced by a different type of corneal surgery. There are several possible replacements, some of them very promising but none yet proven to be safe and reliable.

Everyone in the profession is watching the progress of several groups of researchers who are using lasers to re-contour the outer face of the cornea's central zone—the same small window in front of the pupil that RK leaves untouched. As we have seen, this is the part of the cornea whose curvature really counts. By reshaping the front of it to precise specifications, you theoretically could correct the focus without bending the whole cornea, like RK does. This might work for any kind of error—any degree of myopia, farsightedness, or astigmatism.

This experimental technique, called "laser-shaving", "photo-ablation", or "LRK" (for Laser Refractive Keratoplasty), uses the new Excimer laser, which can vaporize corneal tissue without scorching the adjacent cells. This astonishing feat makes it possible to create a new corneal surface of healthy, clear tissue, which the ever-enthusiastic epithelium can grow back over.

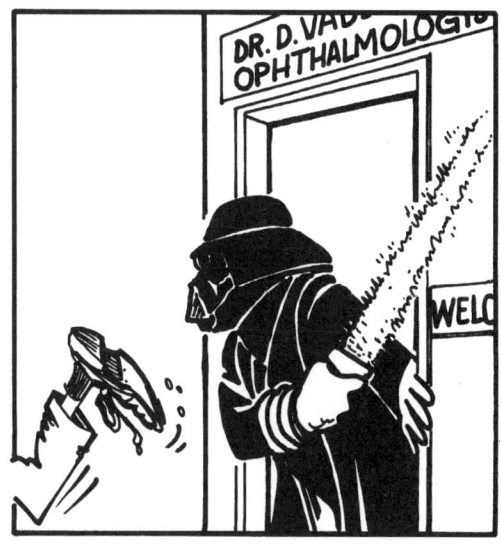

Don't Sell the Bausch & Lomb Stock

Whether or not it will work satisfactorily is what we would all like to know and hope to find out some time in the Nineties, hopefully the early ones. It sounds somewhat horrendous: blasting away part of the vital central window of sight! In this crucial zone even the slightest scarring or haze would be unacceptable, unlike the peripheral area where RK leaves its mark. Also, in order to shave away part of the cornea's thick stroma layer, the laser must first destroy not only the epithelium "skin" but also the thin layer just beneath it called Bowman's Membrane—which, unlike the epithelium, will not immediately grow back. Can the cornea stay healthy without it? Probably—but probably isn't good enough. One disaster in a hundred will be too many. The results with monkeys have been promising, and now tests with people are beginning, but as of now no one can say what the outcome will be.

Suppose Laser-Shaving *Does* cut the Mustard

If this technique works it may eventually replace RK, because it will have several major advantages: no deep cuts that might weaken the eye to blunt trauma or cause fluctuation, no chance of perforation, and above all, it is hoped, no "predictability problem". The laser will be controlled by a computer which is also wired to a curvature-measuring system, so the effect of the operation will be monitored even as it is being performed.

Laser Refractive Keratoplasty has incredible potential—if it works, it could become the standard solution to most refractive errors. Still, it probably will not be widely available for at least ten to fifteen years. The technical difficulties in controlling eye movement and monitoring the cornea's shape while you remodel it are awesome, and it may be necessary to combine the lasering with more conventional surgery to prevent the loss of Bowman's membrane. It could turn out to one of those breakthroughs that are right around the corner forever, but it is a factor to consider if you are contemplating RK, and are in no hurry.

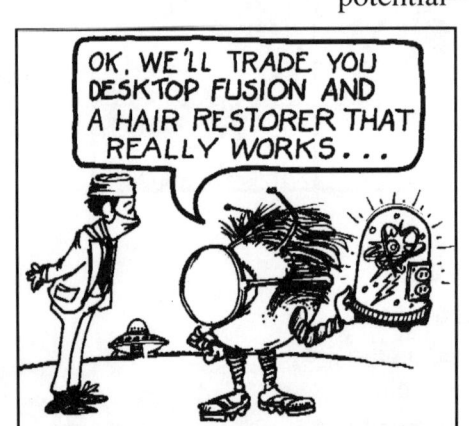

Built-In Contact Lens

Another approach to changing the cornea's shape is to fasten a disc of corneal tissue onto the front of it, an operation called epikeratophakia which is currently used both for high myopia and for extreme farsightedness. At present, donated human tissue is used, but before long a synthetic material will probably be developed which could make this operation much more predictable. Dr. Marguerite MacDonald, a leading refractive-surgery researcher and part of the team at Louisiana State University that developed epikeratophakia, believes this will be the wave of the future for high myopia and farsightedness.

It is also possible to implant a clear plastic lens within the cornea. To install this "intracorneal inlay", the surgeon must make an incision in the outer periphery of the cornea, split the corneal layers, pry them apart, and insert the plastic lens between the separated layers. Tricky! For at least the next decade, it seems unlikely that the intracorneal inlay will be the ideal solution, except in special cases—for example, patients with albinism could benefit greatly from tinted implants.

Belt Tightening

Here's another new idea: an adjustable plastic ring, buried in the peripheral cornea. This can be implanted without touching the central area; only the outermost cornea must be tampered with. Once the ring is installed, the surgeon can either expand or constrict its size—expanding the ring will stretch the cornea flatter, reducing myopia; constricting it will make the central cornea bulge outward, correcting hyperopia.

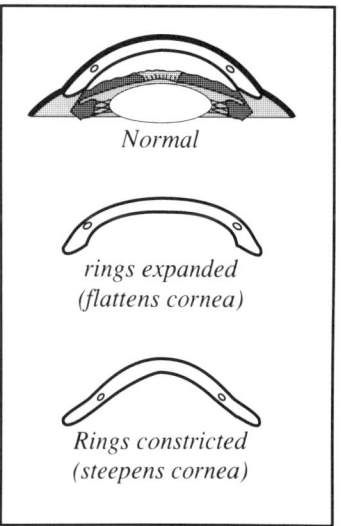

Normal

rings expanded (flattens cornea)

Rings constricted (steepens cornea)

Sounds enticing. Not known yet: does it weaken the cornea? And will it remain in place, or will the cornea eventually eject it?

Move Over, Luke Skywalker

The "laser-shaving" development is the one that has the eye-care community on the edge of its seat. The possibility that every nearsighted, farsighted or astigmatic patient will be completely corrected in a few minutes by a laser beam hooked to a computer—possibly in a series of visits to the ophthalmologist—has mind-boggling implications for the eyewear industry, and for the millions of eyewear-dependent people. If America can maintain its position in the forefront of this research, we may be the first post-eyewear country.

Whichever lines of research turn out to be successful, many readers who choose not to proceed now with RK or another refractive operation will want to keep informed of the progress. That way they'll be in a position to make use of the right procedure as soon as it has been perfected and proven to their satisfaction.

Great Books your Library Won't Have

You may also have questions about the current options that we have failed to answer here. Most can be answered by your doctor, but you might want to do some more reading.

There are several books written by surgeons for use by other surgeons, and having read this one you will be able to follow them. Some of the best are published by a company named SLACK Incorporated in New Jersey. The most up-to-date (as of this writing) is *Refractive Corneal Surgery,* edited by Dr. Donald Sanders and others, with contributed articles by many of the best refractive surgeons, including Doctors Michael Deitz, Robert Hoffman, Herbert Kaufmann, Marguerite McDonald, Spencer Thornton, James Salz, Richard Lindstrom, Richard Villasenor and others.

Other excellent SLACK books include *A Text of Radial Keratotomy* and *Radial Keratotomy: Surgical Techniques.* Yet another fine work on refractive surgery is *Understanding Radial Keratotomy,* by Dr. Ronald A. Schachar and associates. Prof. Benjamin F. Boyd's beautiful book, *Refractive Surgery With the Masters,* describes and illustrates many operations and is very up-to-date. Dr. William Ellis has written a book with an emphasis on astigmatism called *Radial Keratotomy and As-*

tigmatism Surgery.

Almost any experienced RK surgeon will have most of these books; whether he will let you borrow them without leaving your firstborn for collateral is another matter. Offer to leave a security (these books average around a hundred dollars apiece) and promise to return the book within a few days.

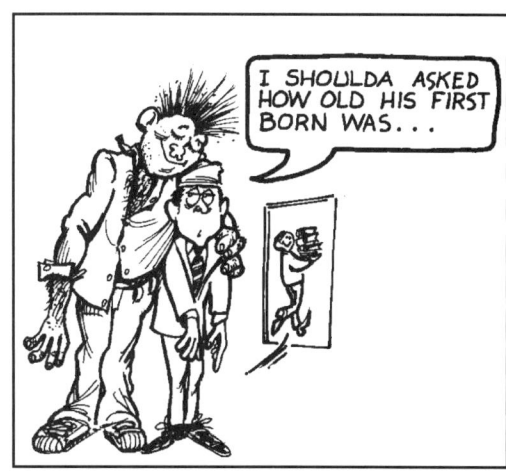

Keen 'Zines

There are half a dozen magazines that publish papers on these developments. One of the best is *Refractive & Corneal Surgery*, the journal of the International Society of Refractive Keratoplasty. It is also published by the SLACK people, and costs $70 a year (6 issues). Exciting developments are covered in every issue; you would probably keep a fairly solid grasp of the state of refractive surgery if you read it and nothing else. SLACK's address is 6900 Grove Rd., Thorofare New Jersey 08086.

The American Journal of Ophthalmology publishes an article or two on refractive surgery each month, and every ophthalmologist has a pile of these in his office. Sometimes he'll let you wade through them in search of articles that interest you. There will probably be copies of *The Journal of the Keratorefractive Society* in that pile, too, which are full of great papers. *Ophthalmic Surgery, Annals of Ophthalmology, Contact Lens Forum, Journal of Cataract and Refractive Surgery, Ophthalmology Times, Ocular Surgery News* and several other periodicals also cover these new procedures. A good university library is an even better source than your doctor's office, of course. Bring a pocketful of change for the copy machine.

If Only Ophthalmology Really Mattered, Like Di's Hairstyle

Sadly, you will get little help from the popular media. The media have barely reached the point where they can clearly report what was known about RK ten years ago, let alone the current status. They milked it's amazing-new-discovery angle for awhile, then tried to find a foolish-yuppie-operation angle, and when that didn't pan out they gave up on it completely. To learn anything really worth knowing, you must seek knowledge aggressively in the non-popular press—but if you do seek, you shall indeed find.

Your research may be frustrating at first as you find that the experts rarely agree about anything new. It takes years for a consensus to evolve. But you will soon identify writers who are rarely far from the mark, and patterns of truth will begin to emerge. Just remember: the first article you read on a given subject cannot be taken for gospel. Look for confirmation, and don't be surprised if you sometimes find contradiction instead.

There's Always Some Disagreement

Almost every field of medicine has its controversies, with some researchers expounding new theories, others defending old doctrines, still others attempting to reconcile the two. In fact, your study of refractive surgery may be valuable training for the future: should you someday have a major medical problem, you will have experience at feeling out the boundaries of knowledge, and be able to judge wisely when the first doctor you talk to is completely contradicted by the second. (This drives

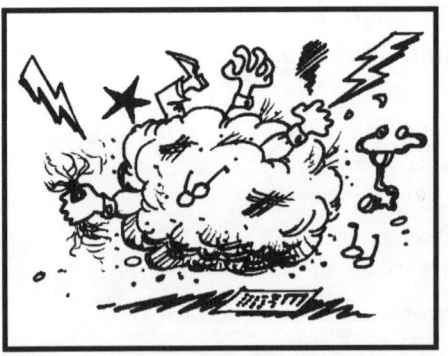

patients crazy, but it's better than the alternative: all the experts in agreement and all dead wrong.) To even the best of doctors you are one of many patients, while to yourself you are the soul and center of the universe. If you keep researching and consulting, you will find the truth.

The Patient's Obligations

It seems to me that those who benefit from RK and other new advances should try to contribute a little to further research. Tell others about what you've learned. Consider investing in the companies that are developing new instruments. Encourage young people to enter this exciting field—for an intelligent and energetic person, the challenge and potential are fantastic. Sign up as an organ donor, or join a service club (like the Lions) that fights blindness. Urge your local press to cover these things better—if the whole field of ophthalmology got as much ink as Mick Jagger, it would be revolutionary.

But first, read the appendices—they're for anybody who wants to keep a set of eyes in good working order.

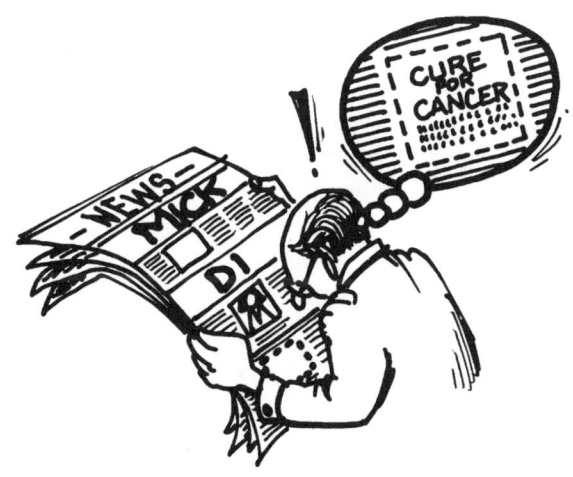

Fifty Million Need Glasses to Read: This has Gone Farsighted Enough

appendix A

Farsightedness, like nearsightedness, is named for its most positive feature. But where the nearsightee really can see nearer than the 20/20 fellow, the farsighted person cannot see any farther, and in fact will lose distance focus as the middle-age vision change, presbyopia, comes along. Farsightedness (also called "hyperopia" or "hypermetropia") is a royal pain and gets worse with time, making presbyopia set in sooner and cause a blurrier near-vision than it does for non-hyperopes.

Farsighted (hyperopic) people need a way to increase the eye's focusing power, rather than decrease it as RK does for the myopic eye.

Also in the market for a safe, predictable eyepower-boosting procedure are many of the older 20/20 people, who, having lost the ability to accommodate for focusing on near vision, would like to have one eye made permanently stronger for reading. These are people who employ "contact-lens monovision" (a contact in one eye for reading) or would if they weren't bedeviled by dry eyes or other problems.

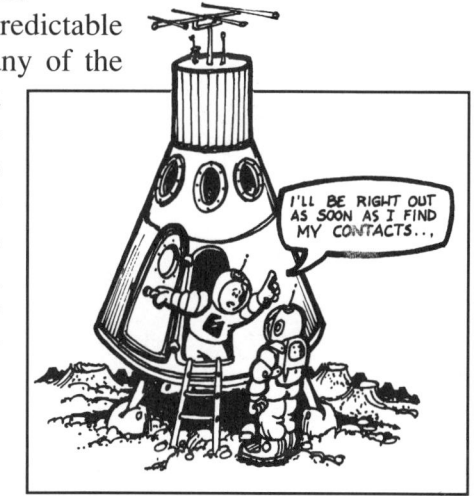

Certainly there are tens of millions who would welcome a refractive surgery for cranking up the focus in one eye or both. If you are such one, it's time to start monitoring the progress in refractive surgery for hyperopia. This has been one of those "We can put a man on the moon but..." situations for long enough.

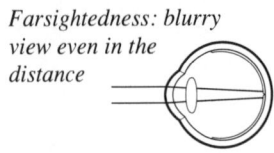
Farsightedness: blurry view even in the distance

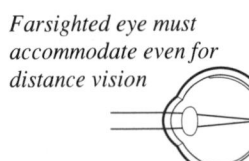
Farsighted eye must accommodate even for distance vision

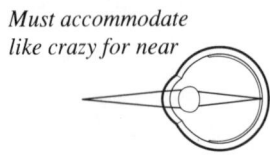
Must accommodate like crazy for near

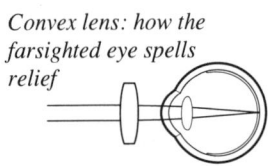
Convex lens: how the farsighted eye spells relief

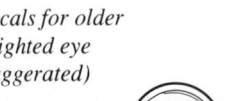
Bifocals for older farsighted eye (exaggerated)

The Underpowered Eye

The farsighted eye is usually a little too short from front to back, so that the image is not quite in focus when it hits the retina. Sometimes the cornea is to blame: it's a bit too flat, and doesn't focus the image strongly enough, with the same result. Either way, farsightedness can be corrected if the cornea can be steepened precisely.

The advantage of farsightedness over myopia is that accommodation, which can't help with myopia, comes to the farsighted person's rescue. The lens thickens up and focuses the image.

For close-up vision, accommodation has to work even harder.

If you're farsighted, you're accommodating all the time without knowing it, unless it starts giving you headaches or eyestrain, which will provoke you to get some plus-powered, convex glasses.

As you get older you lose the ability to accommodate, just as the 20/20 folks and the nearsighted people do. But whereas the 20/20 folks can still see far unaided, and the nearsighted ones can still see near, the farsighted will need glasses for both near and far. They'll usually wear bifocals with a stronger segment for near.

Farsighted people are actually one of the most misunderstood minorities: they have frequently been thought to be "slow learners" because they can't read comfortably. The farsighted child can read, but only by accommodating strenuously—just as the 20/20 person can read a page two or three inches from his nose if he has to.

Nowadays many farsighted children are correctly diagnosed, and glasses are prescribed. But by the time this is done, the child may already have fallen behind, and developed a strong negative association with reading. Also, farsighted children are sometimes uncomfortable with full-correction glasses, because they are used to accommodating for distance vision—that is, their eyes' lenses are in the habit of doing some work even to see far, and don't want to quit accommodating. So the optometrist may feel obliged to prescribe less than a full-powered correction, at least for a while.

The Unseen Error

Mildly farsighted kids sometimes grow up and go clear to middle age without glasses, because for most purposes accommodation can compensate for hyperopia during the first four decades of life. Only two and a half diopters of extra focusing power are required to focus at, say, 15 inches. The human eye starts life with tremendous accommodation ability. At age ten, you still have about thirteen diopters of accommodation. At twenty you have ten diopters; at 30, seven diopters.

Only at age thirty-eight or thereabouts do you really start to notice that you're slightly farsighted, and have been relying on accommodation for distance vision as well as near. The older hyperope (farsighted individual) is unable focus near or far, and the focus gets worse with the passing years until it stabilizes at about age 65.

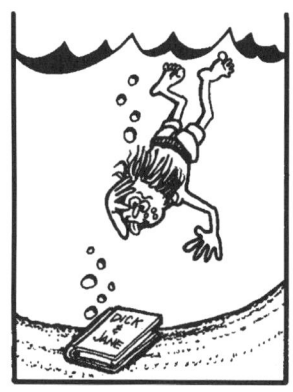

Little kids have so much accomodation, they can almost read under water

Adding some Oooomph

For centuries farsighted people have been fortunate to have convex-lens glasses—plus-powered, light-focusing, magnifying-glass type lenses that deliver the image to the eye already partly focused, and let the poor lens muscle relax. Contact lenses also work fine for many farsighted folks; in fact their convex shape may be more natural and comfortable under the eyelid than the rimmed, concave myopia lenses. Even babies can often wear farsightedness contact lenses, and are thus saved from infantile blindness.

The development of refractive surgery for farsightedness has lagged behind the sensational progress of RK for myopia. Just as it is easier to let air out of a tire than to put more air into one, so it is with the cornea: it has been easier to flatten it than to make it more curved. But now that RK is settling into routine, some of the pioneers are turning their attention to hyperopia, and some promising procedures are being developed. None of them has even a hundredth of the track record that RK has compiled, and possibly not all of the potential hazards have been discovered. Much less has been written than about RK, and there have been no objective PERK-style studies yet. These operations are still experimental, and we won't be able to discuss them and their complications in complete detail. But it seems likely that one or more of the new farsightedness procedures will be widely available within a few years.

Beefing Up the Mildly Underpowered Eye

One method of correcting mild farsightedness is a simple procedure called Hexagonal Keratotomy. It involves RK-type micro-incisions made in the shape of a hexagon around the central part of the cornea, which weaken the cornea and allow the central part to be bowed outward by the pressure of the fluid inside the eye. As the central cornea bulges outward slightly, it becomes more convex and gains a little more focusing power. The change is very slight, perhaps a 5% increase in the cornea's curvature.

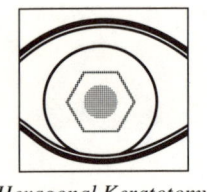

Hexagonal Keratotomy

Hexagonal Keratotomy is relatively simple and fast, like RK, but is harder on the cornea. For one thing, the incisions must be connected to each other, which causes healing to take longer. Also, the nerve endings of the inner cornea are cut, because they radiate inward from the periphery, and the resulting loss of sensation may increase the hazard of inflammation and foreign-body injury, at least until the nerves grow back—probably four or five months.

Probably all of the possible complications of RK that we discussed in Chapter 12 could also occur after Hexagonal RK. (Since all the procedures covered in this chapter are still experimental, we won't be discussing the hazards and other details as thoroughly as we did with RK. If you decide to seek hyperopia surgery, make sure the surgeon tells you all the potential problems.)

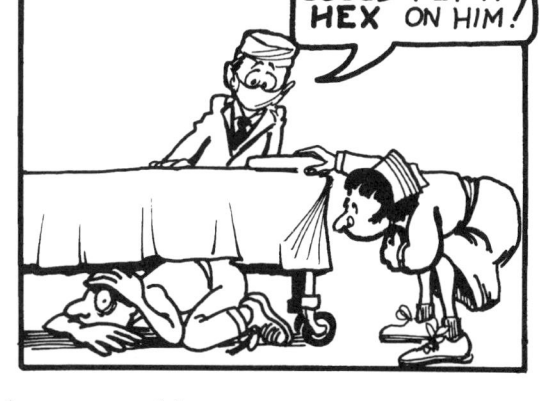

Hexagonal keratotomy works best for low degrees of hyperopia, up to about two diopters. So *if* it compiles a good track record, it may become popular among older people who would like one eye made slightly nearsighted, for reading.

High-Performance Farsight Fixes

For higher degrees of hyperopia, there are two leading candidates. One is a surgical procedure called "HLK" for "hyperopic lamellar keratotomy"—which means "corneal layer separation". The surgeon planes a tiny frisbee of tissue off of the central cornea, which leaves the central cornea thinner and weaker. The thinned central cornea immediately bows outward a bit, under the force of the intraocular pressure. Then the surgeon replaces the frisbee, and sutures it in place. The cornea retains its new, more strongly curved configuration, with more focusing power—the amount of the increase being determined by the diameter of the section that is lathed off and put back on.

This might be a winner. The cornea seems to heal rapidly, and the results appear to be fairly predictable. The cornea is not left any thinner or thicker than before, just more convex. This proce-

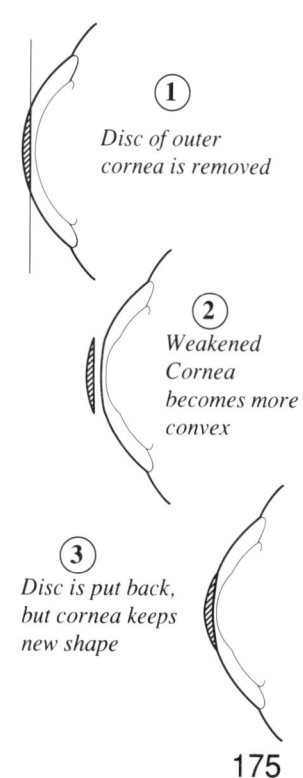

① Disc of outer cornea is removed

② Weakened Cornea becomes more convex

③ Disc is put back, but cornea keeps new shape

dure, pioneered at Colombia's famous Barraquer Institute, is now being developed and performed by Dr. Leo Bores of Scottsdale, Arizona, the surgeon who introduced RK to America. As he did with RK, Dr. Bores waited to amass a meaningful series of results before beginning to teach the procedure to others.

HLK could become a popular means of reducing or correcting moderate farsightedness. However, it is still very new, and demands special training and skill.

From Russia With Love, Again

The other contender for the hyperopia-fixing championship is a completely different kind of surgery: changing the cornea's curvature by altering the molecules of the stroma, its main layer.

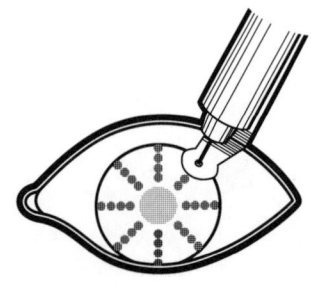

The "Father of RK", Professor Fyodorov, believes that the best solution to hyperopia is to change the molecular structure of the cornea by coagulating it slightly, causing it to shrink a bit in the periphery, thus pulling the central optical zone into a more strongly curved shape. Dr. Fyodorov invented a little heat-probe which uses infra-red radiation as a heat source. He has been using it to perform an operation called "Radial Thermal Keratocoagulation", or RTK, in his Moscow clinic for about four years, and has done over 1000 patients.

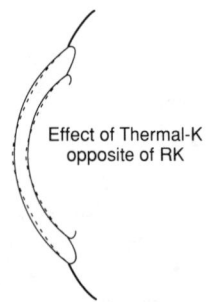

Effect of Thermal-K opposite of RK

The surgeon uses the tiny probe to apply localized bursts of heat, in a radial pattern, to the outer cornea. The stromal tissue around the heated pits coagulates, and shrinks. This is definitely no fun for the cornea, and the pain usually lasts longer than with RK. The foreign-body sensation lasts two weeks, also much longer than with RK. The whitish scars remain visible for several months afterward, before they slowly fade away.

It's not certain whether the thermal approach is a good way to re-do overcorrected RK operations, because the heat may seperate the RK incisions. But Hyperopic Thermal Keratocoagulation could be very useful to correct ordinary farsightedness, and for correcting one eye of an older person for reading. Because it is so new and powerful, it will not be widely accepted until a substantial series of American patients have obtained good results, and the procedure is proven to be safe. The Alcon Corporation is setting up a very thorough and rigorous trial program for the procedure; Dr. Albert Neumann of the Neumann Eye Institute in DeLand, Florida is among the participating surgeons. Many doctors and potential patients will be watching the results of the Alcon study.

Mega-Farsightedness

There is an extreme type of farsightedness, called "aphakia", which occurs when the eye's natural lens—the flexible transparent button that provides 20% of the eye's focusing power, and also provides accommodation—is absent. This lensless condition used to be the fate of all cataract patients: after the clouded lens (cataract) was removed, they were left extremely farsighted, lacking about 13 diopters of power. Today, nearly all cataract patients get an artificial intraocular lens (I.O.L) implanted as part of the surgery, but there are some who don't—including some children with juvenile cataract.

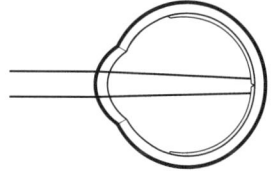

Aphakia: No Lens. Results in extreme farsightedness.

Several operations have been developed for such intense farsightedness, including variations of the keratomileusis and epikeratophakia procedures we discussed in the chapter on high myopia. The "epi" procedure for mega-farsightedness, in fact, seems much more promising than epi for myopia, and is proving to be a godsend for many children who would otherwise be almost blind during crucial formative years.

Readers interested in correcting high hyperopia should read Chapter 17 for research guidance.

Must One Remain a Hyperope? Nope!

The mildly or moderately farsighted person should soon have several refractive-surgery options. None is very well tried or proven yet in America, and only a few surgeons have performed a large number of hyperopia procedures. The most eager patients may be able to consider going ahead soon—hexagonal keratotomy may turn out to be a reasonable procedure for less than +2 D, while for higher degrees of farsightedness perhaps the hyperopic lamellar keratectomy or the thermal-K will turn out to be the way to go.

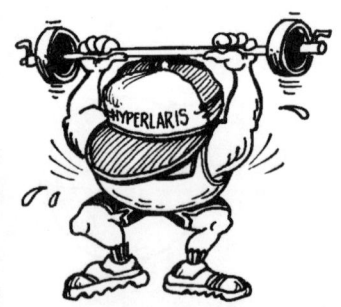

Keep Your Shirt (and Glasses) On a Bit Longer

Since hyperopia correction is improving at a such a ripsnorting pace, most farsighted people will want to wait another year or three, and see which procedure wins the greatest approval—see chapter 17 to find out how to monitor these developments. Hopefully you will be able to escape farsightedness in the near future.

Two Cheers for Glasses and Contact Lenses

appendix B

It will be many years before the external eye-aid is completely phased out, and most readers will be stuck with glasses or contacts for a while longer. In keeping with our aim of being realistic and helpful, here's a few useful facts.

An Ism We Need: the Refractionist

The variety of glasses and contacts available today is mind-boggling. Whether you're near-sighted, astigmatic, presbyopic or any combination of the above, there is probably a pair of glasses and/or contacts that will suit you. But unless you are very easy to please, you need a good refractionist to help you find them.

There are several ways that your glasses can be wrong for you, and some of these mistakes are not obvious even to an expert. If left uncorrected these problems can cause headaches, tension, eyestrain and otherwise take the fun out of life. As we'll see, contacts can foul you up in even more ways, with more serious consequences. So don't buy eyewear like shoes off the rack. Use a good refractionist, usually an optometrist or an ophthalmologist, every time you buy new glasses or contact lenses.

Glasses were invented independently by the Chinese and the Europeans, and until recently were almost always convex, to assist the presbyopic eye with near vision. There are too many different types and styles to go into them all here, but in general the best ones have smallish lenses and wraparound temples that hold them firmly in place. The currently-fashionable huge lenses and straight temples are a goofy design, because the

How Glasses Were Invented

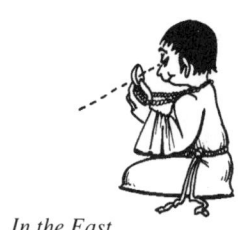

In the East

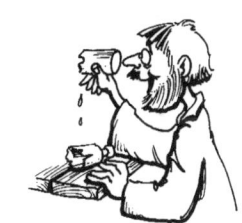

In the West

179

bigger the lens, the thicker it must be at the edges (for myopia), so it is much heavier than a smaller lens. To hold this extra weight the straight temples rely on spring tension, clamping your head between them. Yecch. Also, with myopia the wearer's face tends to appear indented behind the glasses, and larger lenses exaggerate this phenomenon.

All spectacles sold in the United States must be made with hardened glass, which can stand more impact without shattering, and if it is broken will not form such quite sharp, jagged pieces as ordinary crown glass. Better yet is safety glass, but safest of all are plastic lenses, which if they do break—and it takes a hard whack to do the job—don't shatter like glass but break into larger, somewhat blunter pieces. Plastic lenses are also much lighter than glass, and don't fog up so readily.

No, Virginia, There Really Isn't a Baron Von Contact

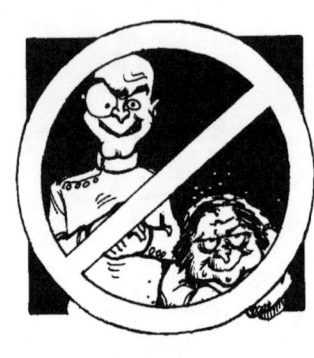

Supposedly, Leonardo da Vinci originated the theory of the contact lens, and not the diabolical Baron von Contact. Plastic contacts have been around for about forty-five years, and are now used by more than twenty million Americans.

The first modern contact lenses were made of the same plastic as the windshield of the Spitfire fighter plane of World War II. When those windshields were shattered by bullets and pieces flew into the pilots' eyes, doctors were astonished to see that the young men's eyes tolerated the plastic fragments instead of rejecting them with inflammation and fever, as expected. This plastic, called PMMA, soon became the material of the first artificial lens designed to be implanted in the eye to replace the natural lens removed during cataract surgery, and also was used to create the first mass-production contact lens, the "hard" contact.

Hard contacts gave clear, crisp vision, but they had plenty of drawbacks. Sometimes, the hard lens would actually warp the cornea over a period of months or years, changing the wearer's refraction in a wildly unpredictable way. If not properly fit, they could cut off the cornea's oxygen supply and cause all kinds of trouble.

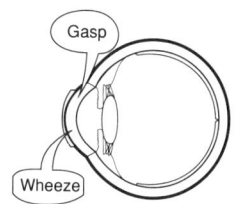

An Eyeful of Trouble

The hard lenses often would deaden the cornea's nerve endings, so early stages of corneal ulcers, inflammations and infections would go unnoticed. The results were sometimes tragic: a report in 1966 on 50,000 contact-lens wearers found nearly eight thousand cases of serious damage, including 14 eyes permanently blinded. It became clear that contact lens wear was a serious business, and the wearer had to be careful.

You Old Softie You

In the sixties came the invention of the soft contact lens, a quantum leap forward in optical technology. The soft contact is porous—in fact, it soaks up more than its weight in water—so it "breathes" well, can be worn longer without suffocating the cornea, is more comfortable, adheres more closely to the eye—and doesn't pop out at every opportunity. The vision is slightly less sharp, but still good. One drawback of the soft lenses: they follow the contour of the cornea, so they can't correct astigmatism like the hard ones can. Also, they are more expensive and less durable—hamhanded fellows like your author are forever tearing them while trying to clean the little monsters.

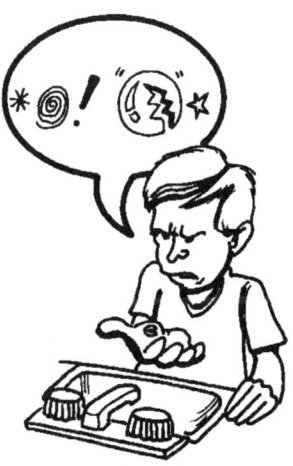

To bacteria, the soft contact lens is a charming country hotel; they happily take up residence and make themselves at home in its warm, wet, spongy interior. So soft lenses must be disinfected regularly, which used to be done by heating. This repeated cooking eventually ruins some lenses, so nowadays chemical means are preferred. Unfortunately, the soft contact absorbs chemicals and builds up deposits, no matter how much you try to keep it clean, and eventually will cause an allergic reaction. A mild reaction causes a red, sore eye; a severe one causes a horrendous swelling called Giant Papillary Conjunctivitis. So doctors advise discarding each lens after about six months of wear—in fact, the new replacement-lens programs offered by companies like Bausch & Lomb may be the best innovations of the decade.

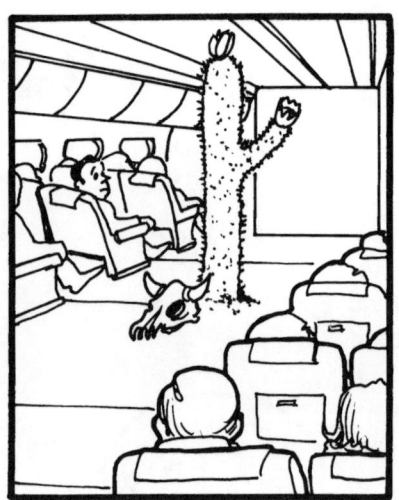

Many people's eyes react to the preservatives that the cleaning and storage solutions contain, such as Thimerosol. So new preservative-free solutions have been developed—which lack the anti-bacteria properties that the preservatives provide, requiring additional anti-contamination steps. Obviously, you have to stay on your toes and in touch with your ophthalmologist once you start developing problems with soft contacts.

Another drawback: if they get too dry in the eye, which can happen in dry weather (including the desert-like atmosphere of an airliner) or windy conditions, or if you leave them in while sleeping, they can shrink and tighten on the cornea. Then they must be moistened prior to removal.

I Tried These Once for Three Hours (But it *Seemed* Like Three Weeks)

For many years, the industry sought a lens which could be left in the eye for three weeks at a time. Today's extended-wear contacts are larger in diameter than daily-wear soft lenses, with a higher proportion of water, so they are more porous and let the eye "breathe" better, which theoretically makes them safer for constant use. However, while some people find them very comfortable, others cannot get used to them, perhaps due to their size.

Also, they can cause trouble if something goes wrong, and the unknowing wearer leaves them in place. So users should get regular checkups.

The current sensation is the disposable lens that you wear for a week or two and then throw away. These will be great for some people who can afford the $500- to $1000-a-year cost, but disastrous for others who will try to save money by leaving them in for too long.

Another innovation is the gas-permeable rigid lens (GPR), which tries to combine the optical perfection and astigmatism-correcting qualities of hard lenses with the breathability of soft ones. Because they breathe so much better, many professionals feel that anyone still wearing the original PMMA hard contacts should switch to GPR's.

For astigmatic eyes, the gas-permeable rigid lenses may be the best solution, although there are also "toric", teaspoon-shaped soft lenses for astigmatism.

Another breakthrough—one that's been breaking through for years without quite reaching the other side—is the bifocal contact lens. Sounds impossible, but it works in theory and for some people it works in practice. The older models relied on the eyelids to hold the lens in place while the eye moved to look through the upper and lower halves, but some newfangled types have a small central button of plus-power, and may allow the eye to focus on both near and far without moving. Another new type of bifocal contact uses the principal of diffraction.

For many older people, monovision works better: they wear only one contact, or a stronger-powered contact in one eye than the other.

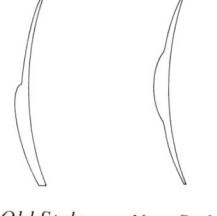

Bi-focal contacts

Old Style   *New Style*

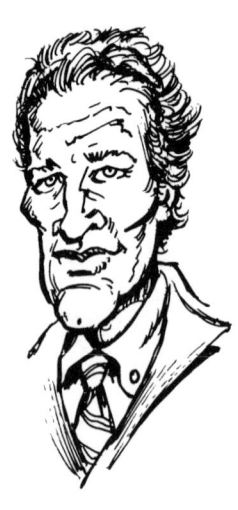

I'd Wear the Blue Ones, But Folks Would Mistake Me for Paul Newman

Recently, colored contact lenses have been introduced, which usually have a clear window in the middle—over the pupil—to see through. At night when the pupil enlarges, the colored coating may get in the way of the wearer's vision, while in bright light the pupil will constrict, revealing the color of the inner iris. Also, they produce a tunnel effect. Still, if I saw a "singles ad" that said "Smashing blonde desperately seeks short, blue-eyed author"...

Why The Baron Likes 'Em

If you wear contacts, remember that there is a foreign body in your eye and you are always at risk. Be watchful, alert, suspicious. The worst that is likely to result from taking your eyes for granted is scarring of the cornea sufficient to require a cornea transplant, which is definitely no fun.

Contact hazards can be divided into infectious and noninfectious types. The noninfectious ones include:

• Lens deposits, especially common with dry-eyed patients. These cause decreased vision and irritation. Lenses must be cleaned or replaced.

• Conjunctivitis, an inflammation of the thin skin that covers the white of the eye and the undersides of the eyelids. One form, Giant Papillary Conjunctivitis (GPC), causes large bumps under the lids, as well as itching and mucus. This is usually caused by an allergic reaction to chemicals that build up in soft lenses.

• The cornea's epithelium can react to lens preservatives, and become cloudy or thickened.

• Neovascularization is an unwanted growth of tiny blood vessels into the cornea, often caused by poor lens fit or overwearing of extended-wear

lenses.
• Hypoxia, or "tight lens syndrome", causes sudden acute pain, decreased vision and other symptoms.

All of these problems require the attention of your eye professional. They usually can be cured in a few days or weeks, and their recurrence prevented. The infectious complications are generally more serious.

Corneal ulcers are the scariest. While they often can be arrested and cleared up with minimal scarring, if untreated these infections can destroy the cornea's clarity (its transplant time) or even spread to the inner eye, resulting in loss of the eye. The symptoms include sudden redness, pain, light sensitivity and tearing. If you experience these you can't get to your ophthalmologist too soon.

There's another infection called acanthamoeba keratitis which causes a ring-shaped fogging of the cornea, and also can lead to a transplant if not treated fast enough. The organisms that cause these infections are found throughout the environment, but may be concentrated in warm wet places like hot tubs. Only by following your eye doc's disinfection instructions to the letter can these little fiends be thwarted.

Another fear with contacts is that long-term damage to the endothelium, that fragile single layer of cells that lines the inside of the cornea. The old hard plastic lenses probably caused more endothelium damage than the new types do, but some ophthalmologists still worry about this problem. Normally, the loss of ten or fifteen percent of your endothelium cells should not cause trouble, but if in senior years you need to have cataract surgery (as about half of us eventually do), that will kill another large fraction of your endothelial cells, and the cumulative loss could be too much, endangering corneal clarity. So try not to "overwear" your contacts. Be kind to your corneas!

Contra-Contact

Some factors which may prevent contact lens use:

Dry eyes, common among older people.

Dry or dusty environments.

Certain diuretic and antihistamine medications (and booze, and coffee) dry out body tissues.

The need to take eyedrops, which can be absorbed by soft lenses.

Pregnancy, which causes many women to stop tolerating contacts.

Arthritis and other physical limitations.

Allergies and seasonal irritations, or other causes of inflammation.

Exposure to cigarette smoke or other atmospheric pollution.

In some people, extreme squeamishness about touching the surface of the eye.

Probably most common of all: inability to make yourself go through all the cleaning and disinfecting rigamarole.

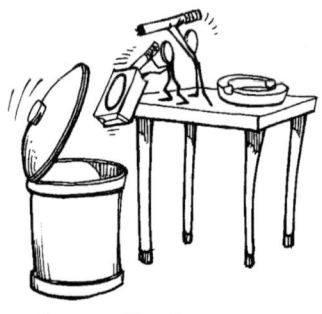

Contacts like cigarettes about as much as the Surgeon General does

A Few Tips for Contact Wearers:

Keep 'em clean. Wash your hands very thoroughly before touching. Dry your hands with air or use lint-free towels. Follow all the steps: you must disinfect the little monsters and also clean them; no single procedure will accomplish both for soft lenses.

Use preservative-free solutions if the Thimerosol burns your eyes, but make sure the doc explains the extra pains you must take to prevent contamination if you don't have the preservative to help out.

Don't wear them longer than you are supposed to. Thou shalt not make an extended-wear lens out of a daily-wear lens by sheer force of will, nor is an extended-wear lens a permanent addition to the eye. As we enter the era of the disposable lens, the incentive to "overwear" them will be greater than ever, and there will be plenty of casualties.

No contact lens will last forever. Soft ones especially become little time bombs, packed with harmful substances. The new fresh-lens programs are revolutionizing contact wear by providing new replacement lenses every three or four months. The new disposable lenses can further reduce the "spoilage" problem if people don't abuse them.

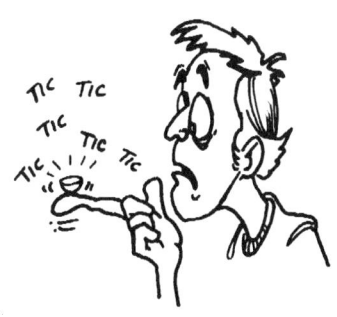

If a lens dries and sticks to your eye, drench it with saline solution and let it moisten up and come loose before you remove it.

Don't wear them in a pool or hot tub unless you like the idea of chlorine being released into your eye for the next forty-eight hours or more. Also, hot tubs are loaded with the bacteria that cause eye infections.

If a soft contact lens mysteriously disappears while you are wearing it, it will be found high up under your upper lid, rolled into a ball. If you can't find it, see your eye pro. It's there. I once had one hide out there for a month.

Follow all instructions, and return to your eye professional for a check-up every six months or so. There's a saying among eye professionals who work with contact lenses: A happy patient is not necessarily a happy eye! Meaning: don't assume all is hunkydory, be suspicious, examine closely.

Contacts are a wonderful invention, and they are being improved all the time. But you can't take them for granted—they are a foreign body in the eye, a tolerated intruder in the most priceless and pristine micro-environment in the world.

There's only one more chapter, about common eye emergencies and how to handle them. If you don't read it you will be blacklisted and never allowed to buy another book of mine.

Eyemergencies

appendix **C**

It could be a couple of decades before you get around to reading another book about eyes, so I feel obligated to provide the following pages of useful information on this one-inch-diameter subject. These facts are really worth knowing, and the first aid summary at the end is worth saving.

Let's start with a scary one: acute glaucoma.

No Exit: Emergency Glaucoma

Chronic, non-acute glaucoma, which troubles about 3% of us, causes the pressure within the eye (intraocular pressure) to increase dangerously over a period of years, and is a very good reason for regular eye check-ups once you pass forty. It can be controlled by medication or surgery 95% of the time, but only after it has been diagnosed. Damage done before diagnosis can't be repaired.

There is also an acute form of glaucoma which happens very suddenly. It usually occurs in only one eye at a time, in which the iris blocks the flow of fluid into the drainage system around the rim of the cornea. Pressure mounts rapidly, causing intense pain in the eye and often in the forehead above it. There may also be blurred vision, weird rainbow effects, a dilated pupil in the affected eye, and sometimes nausea. If you ever experience this, get to a hospital or an ophthalmologist immediately! If the pressure is not relieved within a day the optic nerve will be damaged and vision in the affected eye will probably be lost.

The treatment consists of lowering the pressure with medication, and then tiny surgery with scalpel or laser to remove a small piece of your iris and restore drainage of the fluid. This will prevent further damage, but it won't undo the harm that

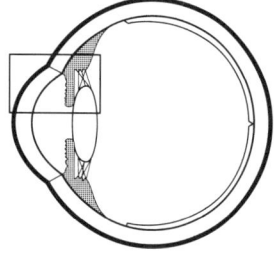

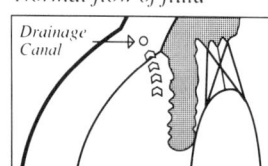
Normal flow of fluid

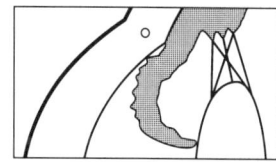
Iris blocks flow

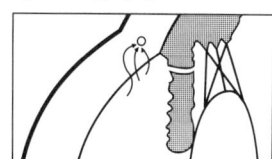
After surgery, flow restored

probably has already been done. So sudden eye pain invokes the Eyefirst Commandment: GET THEE TO THY OPHTHALMOLOGIST OR EMERGENCY ROOM IMMEDIATELY.

Whenever the Commandment is invoked, by the way, the best sequence is a fast phone call to your ophthalmologist, agreement with him or her on where you'll meet (probably his office or an emergency room) and then the drive, with someone else at the wheel. Any emergency-room doctor can usually stabilize the situation, but it's best to get a genuine ophthalmologist ASAP.

Unusual Eye Redness? Don't Play Doctor

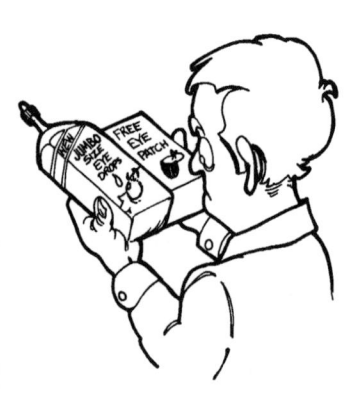

Every eye doctor has seen patients who played doctor and regretted it. Having noticed that one eye was unusually bloodshot, they treated the condition with over-the-counter eyedrops, only to have it come back with a vengeance—because it wasn't caused by smog or dust or other humdrum hazards of modern life, but by something more sinister: acute glaucoma, infection of the lining of the eye or eyelid, corneal infection, severe foreign body trouble, or even endophthalmitis. If you have a red eye, see an ophthalmologist, not a drugstore cashier. We're talking Commandment here.

Foreign Bodies

The corneal epithelium is riddled with nerve endings thick as blades of bluegrass in a Kentucky lawn, so when something gets in your eye, you know it. Usually, the blinking and tear-flooding provoked by the irritation are enough to wash out the offending particle. If not, it will usually be caught under the upper lid, and can be removed by doubling the lid over and fishing it out with a sterile swab or a corkscrew of tissue paper.

Sometimes the particle will be lodged on the

cornea, possibly embedded in the epithelium or even deeper. If so, leave the eye closed—patch it if necessary, but without putting any pressure on it—and head for your eye doc's office. Iron particles can be especially troublesome because they rust rapidly and may stain the cornea.

If you get a foreign body out of your eye, but not before that 5-cell-thick epithelium has been scratched, it will usually heal completely within 24 to 36 hours. Occasionally there may be a more serious corneal abrasion which will begin to hurt more a day or two after the initial problem. When this happens—you guessed it, see your eye doctor. Such abrasions can lead to serious corneal ulcers if left untreated.

Sometimes a foreign body is driven right through the cornea or sclera (white part of the eyeball) into the eye, usually a tiny metal sliver. This happens most often when hammering nails or other metal without protective goggles. Often the immediate pain will go away, leaving you thinking that whatever it was that you got in your eye has been flushed out, when in fact you now have a foreign body inside your eyeball, sure to cause trouble. When in doubt, have the ophth check it out—that slit-lamp gives a great view of the inner eye, like shining a flashlight into a darkened aqarium. And make it a habit to use protection!

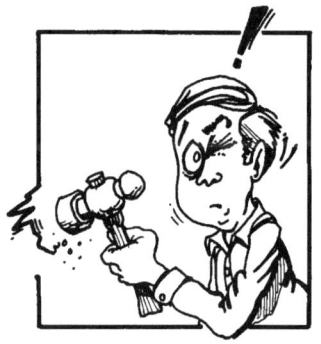

Horror Story: Chemical Burns

Acids and alkali compounds can be very harmful to the eye, especially alkalis. Most types of plaster and cement are alkaline. Many industrial cleansers and solvents, and all drain-opening products, contain enough alkali to blind you. Acid burns the surface but is soon neutralized, while alkali keeps eating away until it is removed.

Never pour these chemicals without first putting on goggles! Don't even buy them without first buying a cheap pair of plastic goggles. If you do splash such a chemical in your eye, get a hose or a faucet *immediately* and hold your burning eye open while you let the water run.

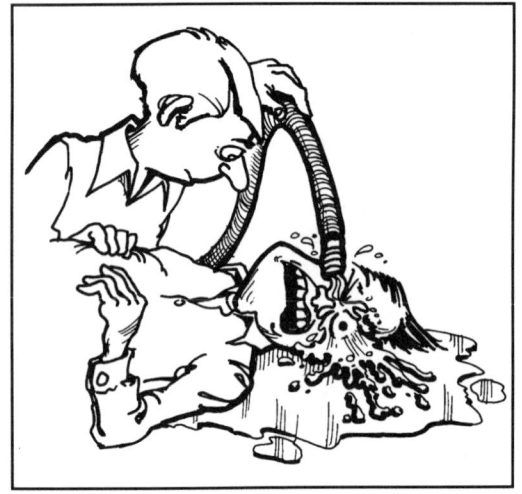

Don't stand there hollering or allowing people to look at your eye, start irrigating it *right away* and don't stop for at least fifteen to thirty minutes. It's best to look to one side, so your cornea isn't directly facing the pressurized stream from the hose. And don't let the chemical run into the other eye!

If solid particles of plaster, lye or other chemical are in your eye, you may stop long enough to remove them with a cotton swab, trying not to scratch the cornea. Then wash, wash, wash. When you have finished irrigating, apply a clean dressing and seek immediate medical attention. Don't rub the eye. Following these instructions may save your sight—even if your cornea is badly scarred, vision can probably be restored through a corneal transplant if you washed the eye soon enough and long enough to prevent deeper destruction.

There are 5,000 Americans waiting for corneas to be available. Please fill out this form and carry in your wallet!

DONOR CARD — EYE BANK ASSOCIATION of AMERICA

In the hope that I may help others, I, the undersigned, being of sound mind and over age 18, wish to make the following anatomical gift at the time of death under the provisions of the Uniform Anatomical Gift Act.

I give: ☐ Any needed organs or parts.   ☐ Eyes only.
☐ Only the following organs/tissues _____

signature _____

witness _____

witness _____

Here We Go Again: Blunt Trauma

Okay, we've already discussed blunt trauma in Chapter 11, in connection with the potential weakness of the post-RK eye. But let's look at it once more, briefly.

A "black eye" is no joke. Many of the potential results can take many years to become apparent. A study in New Jersey showed that one fifth of professional fighters had serious eye problems—these were young men still in the ring; no telling how many more of them will develop trouble later in life.

Possible results of a hard blow to the eye: split or torn cornea or eyeball; ruptured posterior globe or "blowout fracture" of the eye's fragile bony housing; torn or detached retina; hemorrhage; inflammation within the globe or the anterior segment. Blood clots may form within the eye, and the cornea may be stained if the pressure is elevated. The trabecular meshwork may be injured, resulting in glaucoma, and the lens may be injured, resulting in cataract—sometimes many years after the injury.

So be careful out there! Stop beating people up. Be careful with lawnmowers—I find that if I avoid fertilizing or watering my lawn I only need to mow it twice a year, a sacrifice I gladly make in the name of safety. Important: keep kids away from your lawnmower! Their eyes are much closer to the line-of-fire. Wear your seat belt, and be sure to buckle the kids down.

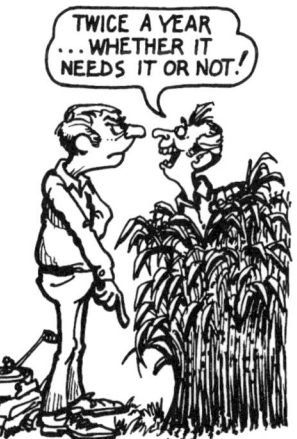

Wear Safety Goggles!

Unless nobody around your pad ever mows a lawn, uses woodworking tools or pours corrosive cleaners, there should be a pair of goggles within reach. If not, get some today! Also get some sport glasses. Even plastic sunglasses are better than nothing for tennis, for example. If you do suffer a hard blow to the eye, don't assume that the "shiner" is the only cost of it—there could be invisible damage. See your ophthalmologist.

Blinded by the Light: Snowblindness, Welding-flash Burn, Eclipse Blindness

Snowblindness, like sunburn, is a situation in which your nerve endings don't get mad, they get even. Rather than hurting immediately, they wait until it's too late for you to do anything to help, and then clobber you. It is actually the cornea and the conjunctiva, the thin skin over the white of your eye, that get sore from the intense light and give you swollen-shut eyes the next day. In my northern state it's a real problem; the Eskimoes invented the first sunglasses centuries ago.

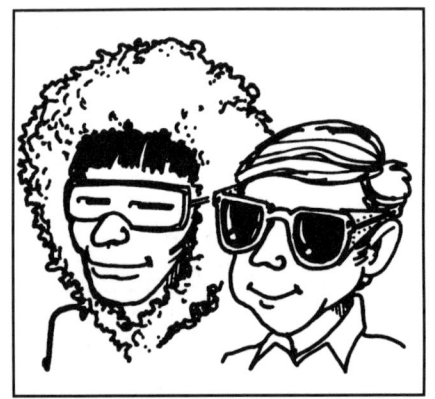

"Instant snowblindness" happens if you look at the arc of a welder for more than a split second: the intense light burns the corneal epithelium and the conjunctiva, and you pay the following day. But no lasting damage is likely to be done.

Not so with the eclipse. Looking at one does no harm to the conjunctiva, but it can severely damage the retina, because the searing light of the sun's corona is focused to a tiny hot pinpoint on the sacred central part of the retina, and literally fries it. "Eclipse blindness" leaves you unable to see what you are looking at, with only peripheral vision remaining. No wonder primitive tribes dreaded this phenomenon! Always be sure of where your children are, and who they are with, during an eclipse.

Indemenace Day

Also know where your children are on the Fourth of July. My brother has just told me of a neighbor's boy being blinded by fireworks this past Fourth—that's just heartbreaking. It's a bitter fact that this heroic date has become an annual festival of juvenile blindness, causing over a thousand cases of severe eye inury each year. It's the flying debris that does it, often from what you think is a safe distance. How many little children can really be trusted to handle such deadly toys?

Better to Angle 'em Off Than Have to Fish 'em Out

Dr. Grendahl points out another hazard familiar to all ophthalmologists who practice near bodies of water: fishhooks! The fishhook actually is a living thing with but one desire: to snag, often on a bush across the creek. When you yank the line and pop it loose, it angrily comes flying right back home to Papa. So wear polarized sunglasses when you fish—they cut glare off the surface and make the fish easier to see (if there are any) and they protect your eyes from getting "tackled".

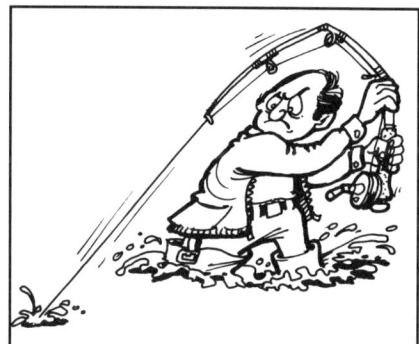

It seems that this world keeps getting more interesting and more dangerous every year—it might be nice if you could leave one eye in a safe-deposit box instead of having to take them both along everywhere you go. New hazards arise regularly: the airless paint sprayer, for example, can put out an eye in a second, yet operators hate to wear goggles because they get covered so quickly by overspray. Drugs like LSD make people lose their common sense and simultaneously inspire them to have wonderful new ideas, like how lovely the sun is to stare at.

There are many eye diseases and problems that I haven't covered, some of which benefit from early diagnosis. Have eye exams more regularly as you get older, especially if you're highly myopic or diabetic, or if there's a family history of eye trouble. Everyone should have a regular ophthalmologist—they really are fun people, often very lively and talkative types who enjoy answering questions. They see your eyes as priceless high-tech instruments which must not be taken for granted, and that's a point of view well worth exploring. Imagine owning a camera worth more to you than all your other property: such in fact is the case.

Hey, you're almost finished! Just read this short, handy summary, suitable for cutting out and putting where you can find it with one eye shut.

Eye First Aid Review

Chemical Burns: Have the victim lie down, if possible, and hold his eyelid open as you pour water continuously over the eye, eyelid, and face. Use a hose, a bucket, a pitcher, anything. Don't let the chemical get into the other eye. Don't rub the eye. Ignore the patient's complaints; he'll thank you later for nearly drowning him. Keep flushing for half an hour if you can—fifteen minutes at least. Cover with a clean dressing, and get to a doctor immediately. If you go to an emergency room, try to have an ophthalmologist meet you there.

Intense pain in one eye, usually accompanied by facial pain (in the forehead over the eye) and general sick or nauseous feeling: Go to eye doctor immediately. Could be acute glaucoma.

Unusual Redness: Don't dose yourself with eyedrops. See a doctor. Many possible causes, some potentially disastrous.

Blunt Injury: ice pack or cold compress to reduce pain, bleeding and inflammation while you head for the doctor's office. Don't put any pressure on it.

Foreign Object Driven Into Eye: Don't let victim rub the eye. Have victim lie down if possible. Wash your hands before you examine victim's eye. Cover both eyes with sterile compress—this will stop all eye motion—and get the victim to an ophthalmologist.

Small Particle In Eye:

1. Pull upper lid down over lower lid. In a few seconds, eye will start to water, and particle may be flushed out.

2. If that fails, flush the eye gently with water from a squeeze bottle—contact-lens solution works great—or medicine dropper.

3. If particle remains, look under the lids. Upper lid can be "everted" by placing a cotton swab or similar item over it, and pulling the lashes out and up over the swab. If you see the particle, use the corner of a wet cloth or tissue to remove it.

4. If you can't get the particle out, or if it seems stuck to the cornea, or any damage seems to have been done, cover both eyes and take patient to the ophthalmologist's office or emergency room.

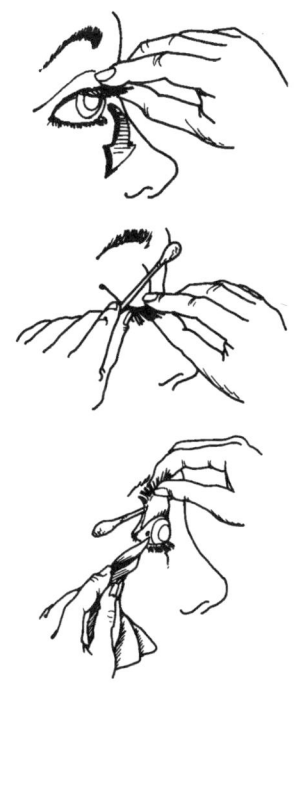

Thanks for reading this last, unasked-for chapter. I hope you enjoyed my book, which is being displayed as proof that with a word processor, any idiot can write one. Be careful, and watch out for the kids—they are hardly ever careful. You've been a great reader, and I hope these chapters will be of help to you.

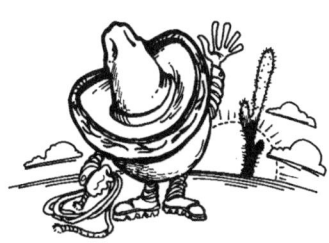

RK Checklist

appendix **D**

Here's a short summary of important steps in the RK process. It leaves out a lot and it's no substitute for reading the whole book, but it might help keep things fresh in your memory.

Pre-operation:

Read all of this book, and decide if you're interested enough to spend about $75 on an eye exam. Really you should have a check-up anyway.

Find a good RK surgeon for the complete exam and conversation. Make sure a cycloplegic test is included. Ask the doc to simulate presbyopia for you as it will be if you're 20/20, and as it will be if you're still nearsighted. Also ask for simulations of imperfect results. Discuss your hopes of monovision and your concerns about avoiding overcorrection and about separate operations, being informed if there's a perforation, choice of anesthetic, etc.

Discuss the odds of success for your particular degree of nearsightedness.

Find out basic cost, and what the additional cost will be if touch-up operation is necessary.

Read all the doc's hand-outs and re-read chapters 11, 12 and 13.

Get a second opinion if desired. Don't rush. Make sure you won't be outraged if you're not in the luckiest 80%.

If you decide to go ahead, decide on a plan. Know which eye is to be done first, what correction doc is shooting for, how many incisions etc.

Stop contact wear and unauthorized drug use, if any, at least 8 weeks prior.

Take antibiotics if doc prescribed same. Follow doc's instructions.

Operation Day:

No booze on op. day. Wash face well. Arrange for ride home and days off from work.

Relax during operation. Expect discomfort and weirdness, don't let them spoil the adventure. Ask doc if it's okay to blink. Remind him which eye we're doing today (a time-honored courtesy of eye surgery). Think about leaves afloat on still waters, and such. Lie still.

Make a friend drive you home and leave you alone. Relax tonight and go to bed early, you earned it.

Post-op:

Doc appointment following day. Don't expect much yet except soreness and light hypersensitivity. Wear sunglasses outdoors.

Take medications prescribed and follow doc's orders.

No unauthorized drugs, especially pot which might cause diminished effect.

Don't panic over temporary visual imperfections but do be alert for infection, especially if perforation occurred.

Hold off on second eye until results with first eye are known, and cycloplegia has been done.

Make sure whether you can keep monovision.

If first eye is still nearsighted, don't pressure the doc into performing a touch-up operation if he's opposed to it. Less is best. Possibly full correction in second eye will make you content.

Follow all anti-contamination and impact-prevention steps. Be careful. Keep all appointments in years to come.

INDEX

Acanthamoeba keratitis, 185
Accommodation
  age and, 17, 37, 173
  definition of, 12
  farsightedness and, 172
  function of, 16-17
  loss of, 137
  nearsightedness and, 20
  in reading, 30-31
  testing of, 18
Accommotrac, 33
Acid burns, 191-192, 196
Age
  accommodation and, 17, 37, 173
  astigmatism keratotomy and, 145-146
  decision for RK and, 119
  radial keratotomy and, 56
AK. *See* **Astigmatism keratotomy**
Alkali burns, 191-192, 196
Anesthesia, 82
Antibiotics, 85, 94
Aphakia, 177
Army
  induction into, 121
  RK research program, 156
Astigmatism
  against-the-rule, 27, 140, 143
  from cataract surgery, 142
  correction of, 22
  definition of, 139
  eyeglass correction for, 140, 141
  with farsightedness, 4, 140
  GRP contact lenses for, 183
  with high myopia, 39-40, 100
  induced, 110
  irregular, 140
  low, 55
  oblique, 140
  overcorrection of, 143
  prescriptions for, 27, 141
  severe, operative strategies for, 144-145
  surgical correction of. *See* **Astigmatism keratotomy**
  uncorrected, 141
  with-the-rule, 27, 140, 143
Astigmatism keratotomy, 40, 72, 85
  age and, 145-146
  predictability of, 146
  surgical correction of, 142-143
Bacterial keratitis, 107
"Barrel-distortion," 39, 73
Bates Method, 32-33
Bifocal contact lenses, 60, 69, 183
Bifocal eyeglasses, 18, 21, 27, 172
Biofeedback device, to correct myopia, 33
Black eye, 193
Blindness
  caused by fireworks, 195
  caused by intense light, 194
  juvenile, 195
  legal, 23, 35
Blood clots, 193
Blowout fracture, orbital, 193
Blunt trauma
  danger of, after RK, 90-91, 107-108, 193
  first aid for, 197
Bowman's membrane, 163

Cataract surgery
  astigmatism from, 142
  risks in, 136
Cataracts
  age-related, 54
  aphakia and, 177
  post-operative, 114
Central zone, 83
Channel theory, 161
Chemical burns, 191-192, 196
Children
  accommodation and, 17
  farsighted, 172-173
  nearsighted, 5
  reading by, myopia and, 29-30
Clear-lens extraction, 136-137, 138
Clear zone, 71
Conjunctivitis, 184
Contact lens(es)
  for astigmatism, 142
  bifocal, 60, 69, 183
  built-in (epikeratophakia), 138, 164-165, 177
  colored, 184
  contraindications to usage, 186

201

extended-wear, 182-183
for farsightedness, 173
gas-permeable rigid, 110, 183
hard, 180-181
hazards of, 3, 184-185
invention of, 34
for one eye, 63-64
post-RK fitting problem, 112-113
risks of, 114-115
safety of, vs. RK, 120
soft, 181-182, 187
usage tips, 186-187
wearing before eye examination, 49-50
Contact-lens monovision, 21, 60, 171
Cornea
adjustable implanted plastic ring for, 165
correction of, in radial keratotomy, 7
curvature of, 45
donation, 192
endothelium, 113-114
epithelium, 43-33, 111
flattening of, by wearing contact lenses, 33-34
focusing power of, 4, 45
individual variations in, 161
laser sculpturing of, 126-127
layers of, 43-44
non-RK flattening procedures, 134-137
role in eyesight, 11
thickness, testing of, 83-83
Corneal layer separation, for farsightedness, 175-176
Coupling, 143
Cycloplegic refraction, 33, 51, 64

Depth perception, 62
Diopters, 25, 35-36, 45
Diplopia, 93, 110-111
Dominant eye, 53-54
Double vision, 93, 110-111
Drugs, 50, 162, 195

Eclipse blindness, 194
Emergencies
blinded by light, 194
blunt trauma, 193
chemical burns, 191-192
eye redness, 190
first aid procedures for, 196-197
foreign bodies, 190-191
glaucoma, 189-190
juvenile blindness, 195
Emmetropia, 19, 25, 95
Endophthalmitis, 106-107
Epikeratophakia, 109, 134-135, 138, 164-165, 177
Epithelium, corneal, 43-44, 111
Eye
anatomy of, 11-14
dominant, 53-54
how it works, 11-17
oval, 22
Eye examination, 49-52
Eye redness, 190
Eyedrops, cycloplegic, 51
Eyeglasses, *See* **Glasses**
Eyelid, droopy, 93

Farsightedness
accommodation and, 172
with astigmatism, 4, 140
astigmatism and, 22
corneal layer separation for, 175-176
description of, 171
hexagonal keratotomy for, 174-175
intense, 177
mild or moderate, 178
prescription for, 27
Fireworks, blindness from, 195
Fishhooks, 195
Flare, 88-89
Fluctuating vision, 90
Focusing, 1, 16-17. *See also* **Refraction**
errors, correction of, 4
near-point, 12
Foreign bodies, 190-191
first aid for, 197
"Foreign body sensation," 87
Fovea, 13, 15, 16

Gas-permeable rigid (GPR) contact lenses, 110, 183
Giant papillary conjunctivitis, 182
Glare, 89-90, 108
"Glare disability," 39
Glasses
ability to read without, 122-123

for children, 5
for farsightedness, 172-173
for moderate myopia, 38
for night driving, 109
prescriptions for, 23, 26, 141
for reading, 17-18
styles of, 179-180
as time-honored solution to myopia, 34
unhappiness with, 2, 3
Glaucoma, 52, 189-190
GPR (gas-permeable rigid) contact lenses, 110, 183

Happiness chart, 102-103
Hexagonal keratotomy, 174-175, 178
Holistic medicine, 32-33
Hypermetropia. *See* **Farsightednes**
Hyperopia. *See* **Farsightedness**
Hyperopic lamellar keratotomy (HLK), for farsightedness, 175-176
Hypoxia, 185

Infection, postoperative, 94
Insurance, radial keratotomy and, 154-156
Intracorneal inlay, 164-165
Intraocular lens implant (IOL), 177
Intraocular pressure, 50, 55
    increased, lowering in emergency glaucoma, 189-190
IOL (intraocular lens implant), 177
I.Q., high myopia and, 129
Iris, 11

Juvenile blindness, 195

Keratitis, bacterial, 107
Keratometer, 53
Keratomileusis, 134, 138, 177
Keratomileusis in situ, 135 <EP>

Laser cornea-sculpturing, 126-127
Laser refractive keratoplasty, 162-164
Laser-shaving, 162-164
Lazy eye, 93
Legally blind, 23, 35
Lens, eyeglasses
    2-diopter, 25
    4-diopter, 25
Lens, natural

function of, 12
removal of, with replacement of artificial one, 137
LSD, 195

Macula, 13, 15, 16
Marijuana, 50, 55, 87
Medical history, 50
Microperforations, 113
"Mini-myope," 37
Minus-form prescriptions, 27, 141
MKM (myopic keratomileusis), 134, 138, 177
Monovision
    contact-lens, 21, 60, 171
    definition of, 59
    disadvantages of, 63
    favoritism for, 68
    toleration of, 61, 62-63
Myopia
    3-D, 36
    2-D, in one eye, 65-66
    advantage of, 59
    with astigmatism, 140
    causes of, 29-30
    in children, 5
    definition of, 1, 2
    degrees of, 35
    description of, 6, 19
    first notice of, 35
    glasses, as time-honored solution, 34
    high, 39, 73, 129
    high, with astigmatism, 39-40
    I.Q. and, 129
    low, 37, 98
    moderate, 38-39, 99
    in modern civilization, 31-32
    overcorrection of, 75
    presbyopia and, 9, 38, 59, 122
    radial keratotomy success in, 98-100, 131-132, 132-133
    refraction, 26
    rough test for, 35-36
    undercorrection, 72
    very-high progressive, 133
Myopic epikeratophakia ("epi"), 109, 134-135, 138, 164-165, 177
Myopic keratomileusis (MKM), 134, 138, 177

Nearsighted, "revenge of," 5, 20-21, 59
Nearsightedness. *See* **Myopia**
Neovascularization, 184-185
Night vision, decreased, 109

Oculis dexter (O.D.), 26
Oculis sinister (O.S.), 26
Ophthalmologist
   active promotion of RK, 152-153
   anterior-segment surgeons, 150-151
   finding one who performs RK,
     149-150
   functions of, 3, 26
   informing patient about RK, 57-58
   inquiries about, 151-152
   performance of Rk by, 147
Optic nerve, 13
Optical zone, 45, 83
Optometrist, 26
Orbit, blowout fracture of, 193
Orthokeratology, 33-34
O.S. (oculis sinister), 26
O.U., 26
Overcorrection, 95, 97-98, 160-161

Pachymeter, 53
Pain, intense eye, first aid for, 196
Patient, obligations of, 169
PERK Study, 42, 109
Phoropter, 51
Photo-ablation, 162-164
Photophobia, 88
Plus-form prescriptions, 141
PMMA, 180
Preoperative planning, 69
Presbyopia
   definition of, 4, 17
   instant, 137
   low myopia and, 37
   nearsightedness and, 9, 38, 59, 122
Prescription drugs, 50
Prescriptions
   for astigmatism, 27
   for eyeglasses, 23, 26, 141
   minus-form, 27, 141
Protective eyewear, 91-92
Pseudomyopia, 33, 51
Ptosis, 93
Pupil, 11
Pus-production, copious, 94

Radial keratotomy
   age and, 56, 119
   alternative surgeries, 162-166
   American technique for, 41-42
   appointment for operation, 8
   books about, 166-167
   candidates for, 54, 69
   career advancement and, 120
   cautious approach to, 74-75, 130
   controversy, 10, 147-148, 168-169
   corneal endothelium and, 113-114
   corneal incisions in, 42, 45-46
   correction of mild astigmatism,
     143-144
   cost of, 153-154, 157
   cutting close to central zone, 71-72
   decision, 7-9, 58, 117-119, 124-125
   depth of incisions, 71, 84-85
   disadvantages of, 115
   dissatisfaction with, 57-58
   effectiveness of results, 162
   first, 41
   four-incision, 75
   future of, 159-160
   improvements in, 125-126, 160-161
   induction into Army and, 121
   insurance and, 154-156
   irrigation of incisions, 85
   learning of procedure, 148-149
   magazines about, 167
   mild myopia as successful result,
     130-131
   for moderate myopia, 38
   news media and, 168
   nomograms for operative
     specifications, 73-74
   on nondominant eye, 67
   number of incisions for, 70, 72
   on one eye, 59, 60-61, 67-68, 93-94
   operative checklist, 200
   operative technique, 80
   outcome, 103, 119
   partial correction of second eye,
     64-65
   patient information on, 57-58
   patient understanding of, 8-9
   plus-or-minus one diopter standard,
     100-101
   possible replacement surgery,

162-163
postoperative period, 8, 80, 85-86, 144, 200
preoperative period, 79, 81, 199-200
prospective patients for, 7
prospective results, 98
protection against infection, 92
psychological aspects of, 56-57
purpose of, 1, 2-3
rationale for, 6-7
re-operation for, 75-76, 96
recovery from, 87
reporting of results, 100-103
results of, 80, 95
reversibility of, 109
risks of. See **Risks of radial keratotomy**
success of, 3, 129
surgical plan, 76-78
on two eyes, 93
vs. contact lenses, 114-115
when to have, 125
why it works, 46-47
Radial thermal keratocoagulation (RTK), 176-177
Redness, eye, first aid for, 196
Refraction
cycloplegic, 33
eyeglass prescription and, 26
measure of, 25
nature of, 14-17
nearsighted, 26
testing of, 50-51
Refractionist, 179-180
Refractive errors, 4
Refractive surgery 1 14 173-174
See also specific surgery
Relaxing incisions, 142-143
Retina, 12-13, 53
Retinal detachment, 136
Retinoscope, 51
"Revenge of the nearsighted," 5, 20-21, 59
Risks of radial keratotomy
decrease in best-corrected vision, 111
decreased night vision, 109
double vision in single eye, 110-111
fluctuating vision, 109
incidence of, 105
infection, 106

long-term fluctuations in vision, 109-110
post-perf precautions, 106-107
postoperative blunt trauma, 107-108
temporary erosions of corneal epithelium, 111
worst that could happen, 106
RK. See **Radial keratotomy**
RTK (radial thermal keratocoagulation), 176-177
Ruiz procedure, modified, 144-145

Safety goggles, 193-194
School myopia, 33
Scleral reinforcement, 133
Sleeping, eye protection during, 92
Slit-lamp microscope, 52
Snellen Visual Acuity Chart, 23-24, 50
Snell's law, 15
Snowblindness, 194
Sports
  participation in, after RK, 122
  protective eye-wear for, 91-92
Stereo-acuity, 62
Steroids, post-operative usage, 114
Sunglasses, 88

T-cuts, 144
Three-diopter myope, 26
Tight lens syndrome, 185
Tonometer, 52
20/15 vision, 23
20/10 vision, 23
20/20 vision, 16
20/200 vision, 23

Undercorrection, 95, 96, 101-102

Vanity, 123-124
Vision
  best-corrected, decrease in, 111
  fluctuating, 109
  long-term fluctuations in, 109-110
Visual acuity testing, 50
Visual axis
  location of, 13, 16
  marking of, 82-83
Visual life cycles, 61

Wandering eye, 112
Welding-flash burn, 194

Glossary

Accommodation: eye's ability to focus on near point by increasing focusing power of the lens. Is lost in middle age.

Anterior segment: front third of eye, including cornea, iris, ciliary muscle and lens.

Anterior Chamber Lens: lens implanted in front of iris to correct refractive error. Also called "Intraocular Spectacles".

Aphakia: absence of eye's natural lens, usually after cataract surgery.

Aqueous: clear fluid behind the cornea. Maintains intraocular pressure.

Astigmatism: refractive error in which the eye's power is not the same in all meridians.

Barrel-distortion: effect of glasses for high myopia. Squares appear barrel-shaped.

Bates Method: controversial holistic approach to improving vision.

Bifocals: glasses with two different-powered lenses, with added power for near vision.

Blind spot: we all have one in each eye, where the optic nerve exits the eye.

Blowout fracture: hard impact to eye can cause it to break through the thin bony floor or sides of the orbit, into one of the nasal sinuses.

Bowman's membrane: very thin layer of the cornea, just under epithelium.

Capsule of lens: elastic membrane around lens.

Cataract: clouding of lens, usually in later years, may require removal of lens. Happens to most of us.

Ciliary body: circular body containing ciliary muscle, which adjusts shape of lens in accommodation. Also produces aqueous fluid.

Clear-lens extraction: procedure for correcting high myopia by removing natural lens.

Concave lens: minus-powered lens for myopia, thinner at center than edges.

Conjunctiva: thin membrane on inner side of eyelids and front of eye, except cornea.

Contact lens: corrective lens that lies directly on the eye.

Contrast sensitivity: measurable visual function, decrease of which may clue doc in to eye problem

Convex lens: plus-powered lens, used for farsightedness and presbyopia.

Cornea: eye's clear front window and most powerful refractive (focusing) surface.

Counts-fingers vision: low level of vision, below 20/400.

Cycloplegic refraction: vision test performed after lens' accommodation has been paralyzed with cycloplegic eyedrops.

Cylindrical lens: lens with more power in one meridian than another, used to correct astigmatism.

D: abbreviation of Diopter.

Descemet's membrane: very thin membrane in cornea, between endothelium and stroma.

Diopter: Unit of measurement of lens power. One diopter equals power needed to focus in one meter (about 40 inches). Two-diopter lens will focus in half a meter, etc. The excess power of the nearsighted eye is expressed as negative diopters (e.g., -2D) because negative-powered concave lens is used to correct it.

Diplopia: double vision. When it occurs in one eye, it's called monocular diplopia.

Glossary

Dominant eye: Favored eye, usually on same side as dominant hand.

Donor cornea, donor tissue, donor graft: from eye bank, donated by one who no longer needs it to one who does.

Emmetropia: condition of the perfectly focused eye, neither myopic nor hyperopic.

Endothelium: layer of cells lining inner face of cornea.

Endophthalmitis: infection within the eye.

Epikeratophakia: surgery involving placement of donor tissue over patient's cornea.

Epithelium of cornea: skin-like layer over cornea.

Eye: oh come on.

Fovea: tiny pit in the center of macula, the hypersensitive part of retina which produces sharp central vision.

Fusion: blending of two eyes' images by brain.

Glare: undesirable hazing of vision due to diffusion of light.

Glaucoma: major preventable cause of vision loss, caused by increased pressure within the eye. Can be slow and chronic, or sudden and acute.

Hexagonal keratotomy: procedure for correcting mild hyperopia.

High myopia: strong nearsightedness, above 6 diopters or so.

HLK: see Lamellar Keratectomy for Hyperopia.

Hyperopia: farsightedness, underpowered eye. Also called hypermetropia.

Induced astigmatism: unintentionally caused by surgery.

Infinity: in visual optics, twenty feet.

Informed Consent form: legal document in which patient states that he is aware of risks and hazards of an operation but consents to it anyway.

Intraocular lens (IOL): plastic lens implanted in eye to replace natural lens removed in cataract surgery.

Intraocular pressure: fluid pressure within the eye.

Iris: pigmented circular curtain behind cornea which dilates or contracts to control amount of light admitted to eye.

Irregular astigmatism: abnormal astigmatism not correctable with glasses.

Kera: Latin for cornea.

Keratitis: inflammation of cornea.

Keratectomy: any surgery in which any part of cornea is removed.

Keratotomy: incision in cornea.

Keratometer: tool for measuring corneal curvature.

Keratomileusis: type of surgery for high myopia (MKM) or hyperopia.

Keratoscope: device for detecting corneal astigmatism.

Lamellar Keratectomy for Hyperopia (HLK): new surgery to cure farsightedness.

Legal blindness: less than 20/200 best corrected vision.

Lens, crystalline: natural lens of eye.

Lens, optical: any transparent peice of material able to bend light in a predictable way.

Lions International: humanitarian organization which performs many services in vision field

Macula: small central disk of retina surrounding fovea which produces central vision.

Manifest refraction: objective test of vision, without cycloplegia.

Minus lens: see concave lens.

MKM: Myopic Keratomileusis.

Glossary

Monovision: ability to see well with two differently-powered eyes, one slightly stronger for reading or near work. Can be achieved through use of contact lenses or RK.

Myopia: nearsightedness, too-strong eye.

Nearsightedness: where have you been?

Ocular: pertaining to eye.

OD: oculis dexter, right eye.

OS: oculis sinister, left eye.

Ophthalmologist: eye surgeon or doctor.

Ophthalmoscope: glorified flashlight for examining interior of eye, mainly retina.

Optical zone, optical clear zone, optic cap: crucial central portion of cornea.

Optician: one who sells glasses and contact lenses from prescriptions provided by ophthalmologists or optometrists.

Optic nerve: major nerve from retina to brain.

Optics: branch of physics concerned with refraction and reflection of light.

Optometrist: "Well-eye doctor", non-medical professional who examines eyes and prescribes glasses or contacts.

Orbit: skull cavity containing eyeball.

Orthokeratology: controversial method of correcting myopia by flattening cornea with contact lenses.

OU: Oculi Uterque, both eyes.

Overcorrection: effect of surgery greater than desired

PERK Study: Prospective Examination of Radial Keratotomy, a clinical trial of RK in 435 patients, funded by the National Eye Institute.

Pachymeter or pachometer: device for measuring cornea's thickness.

Phoropter: device containing huge number of lens simulations, used for refraction testing.

Photophobia: unusual sensitivity to light.

Plano: flat lens with no power.

Plus-sign eyes: found only in dead or unconscious cartoon characters.

Pot: slang for marijuana, a drug which lowers intraocular pressure.

Presbyopia: loss of accommodation ability which usually becomes noticeable by age 45 or thereabouts.

Prosthesis: artificial device or other replacement of missing body part or function

Pseudo-myopia: unintentional accommodation causing temporary nearsightedness.

Ptosis: drooping of upper eyelid. The P is silent.

Pupil: doughnut-hole in the middle of iris.

Radial Keratotomy, Radial K, RK: microsurgical procedure to correct myopia.

Red Eye: common name for conjuctivitis, inflammation of tissues covering front of eye.

Refraction: 1. Optics—bending of light rays as they pass from one medium to another. 2. Test—determination of eye's refractive error ("doing a refraction").

Refractive surgery: any surgical procedure intended to correct focusing (refractive) errors.

Retina: colony of light-sensitive cells lining the interior of the back two-thirds of the eye, which converts visual image to electrical impulses sent to brain.

Retinoscope: hand-held device for measuring refractive error.

Retrobulbar injection: injection behind the eye, into eye muscle. Rarely used for RK.

RK: Radial Keratotomy.

Ruiz procedure: type of keratotomy for astigmatism.

Glossary

Sclera: white of the eye, fibrous globe continuous with cornea.

Slit lamp: microscope for examining front parts of eye.

Snellen chart: eye chart, for measuring visual acuity.

Snellen Acuity: vision according to Snellen chart.

Spectacles: if you didn't know you wouldn't be here.

Stroma: main layer of cornea.

Sutures: surgical stitches.

T-cuts, T-incisions: transverse incisions added to RK to correct mild astigmatism.

Thermal-K, hyperopic: new procedure to correct hyperopia using heat.

Tonometer: instrument for measuring intraocular pressure.

Visual acuity: subjective measure of eye's ability to see.

Visual axis: imaginary line between retinal's central spot, the fovea, and whatever you are looking at.

Visual field, field of vision: extent of area visible to eye as it fixates straight ahead.

Visual Profile: used by some professionals to summarize results of Snellen-acuity, contrast sensitivity and glare disability tests.

Vitreous: transparent, gelatinous mass filling rear two-thirds of eye.

Walletectomy: extraction of funds, usually without anesthesia.

Zonules: radial fibers which connect lens to ciliary body, hold lens in place.

Acknowledgments

My thanks to:

Marvin J. Grendahl, M.D., my own ophthalmologist and patient teacher

James J. Salz, M.D., clear-eyed sceptic, who believed in this project when it counted

Leo D. Bores, M.D., whose courage and energy launched RK in America and whose acerbic comments on my drafts launched me back to the typewriter a time or two

The many others, including Doctors Robert H. Marmer, Michael R. Deitz, Francis Young, Robert W. Miller, Elizabeth R. Vaughan, and Ronald A. Schachar, who answered my questions, and all who have contributed to the body of literature that makes this book possible

Herb King III, virtuoso of the Macintosh and perseverent problem solver, and Bud Root, Alaska's best cartoonist among his other talents

Daisy Hunter Crater, Greg Smiley, Dan Pond, Michael Crater and many others who read and advised

My brother Ted Crater, he of the soaked shoulder

The people at SLACK Inc, whose previous books in this field are a priceless resource

And especially to you for actually reading the darn thing.

About This Edition

This book was written and produced by John Crater, an Alaskan who likes to windsurf and climb the local mountains. John had RK in 1985 after a 25-year hate/hate relationship with myopia, and in 1987 and '88 he spent 18 months of evenings researching and writing this book.

The cartoons were executed by Bud Root, Alaskan artist and caricaturist. The eye drawings are the craftmanship of Herb King III, also of the 49th State. John and Herb designed it and made up the pages on a Macintosh SE with Pagemaker.

The information in the book all comes from MD's, but no single doctor will agree with every point in the book. New knowledge develops all the time, and the book will probably turn out to be wrong on some points. Revised editions are expected. The writer is not an accredited authority on refractive surgery and you must not base any medical decision on this book.